Holistic Approach of Yoga

Holistic Approach of Yoga

Editor

GANESH SHANKAR

Commonwealth

Published under the authority of Dr. H.S. Gour University, Sagar (M.P.)

Holistic Approach of Yoga

Edition **2027**

ISBN : 81-7169-497-7

Published by :
COMMONWEALTH PUBLISHERS (P) LTD.
4831/24, Govind Lane,
Ansari Road, Darya Ganj,
New Delhi - 110002
Ph. : 23272541, 23242541
e-mail : commonwealthpublishers2016@gmail.com

Distributed by :
ARJUN PUBLISHING HOUSE
4831/24, Govind Lane,
Ansari Road, Darya Ganj,
New Delhi - 110002
Ph. : 23272541, 23242541
e-mail : arjunbooks2001@gmail.com

Laser Typesetting by :
Dimple Computers
Delhi

Printed at :
Milan Enterprises
Delhi

Foreword

I am glad that the Department of Yogic Studies, is bringing out the proceedings of the National Seminar on 'Holistic Approach of Yoga for Human Resource Development' which was concluded during Feb., 1997 in our University. It would be an occasion for great satisfaction not only to the learned circles but also the general readers who would expect an absorbing and authentic presentations of the deeper implications of the system of Yoga.

Today, Yoga has become very popular through—out the world as it helps man to develop his mind and intellect leading to realisation of ultimate reality. Particularly, in the world of today, when man is subjected to tremendous stress and strain of life, Yoga can undoubtedly bring peace and harmony. Hence, it has become necessary to reorient our curricula for young students to include Yoga.

I extend my heartiest congratulations to Dr. Ganesh Shankar Giri for his sustained efforts and interest in bringing out this volume. I am fully confident that the present work in the book form will prove useful to the public, inquistive readers of Yoga and Research Scholars alike.

SHIVKUMAR SHRIVASTAVA

Preface

The word "YOGA" signifies functional integration at the highest level of spirituo-psychosomatic development, ensuring not only the health of the body but also experiencing the sense of well being of the senses, the mind and the soul simultaneously. It has, therefore, laid down certain ways and means in the form of various physical and mental procedures to counteract the malicious environmental influences within and without the organism. The holistic approach of yoga or all such yogic practices including *Yamas*—the rules of social hygiene, *Niyamas*—rules of personal hygiene, *Suddhi Kriyas*—purificatory procedures, *Asanas*—postural patterns, *Pranayamas*—breathing exercises, and meditation etc. are prescribed with the purpose of conditioning and/or reconditioning the body-mind machinery so as to extend its range of adaptability and this to achieve a harmonious development of the human personality. Yoga being a subject of varied interests has gained world wide popularity. Recent scientific research trends have shown that it can serve as an applied science in a number of fields such as health and family welfare, medicine and therapy, education, physical education and sports and also as one of the valuable means for self-realization and thereby development of human resources for better performance and productivity in daily life.

Health is a concern of every person. The scope of application of yogic practices for health and fitness has been increasing day by day. Also the therapeutic aspect of yoga has been very popular as an alternative method of treatment of various diseases in modern times. Yoga has been found very much useful for psychosomatic disorders in the present times. Not only that, the aim and objectives of yoga and education are very similar to each other *i.e.* both the desciplines aim at the individual's achievement of all round development or harmonious development of human personality. Therefore, Yoga can be very much useful in the educational process. Further, yogic practices can be used as physiological and psychological procedures for psychosomatic fitness to prevent various injuries in sports activities and help in the rehabilitation of the injured and ill athletes if learnt under the proper guidance and practised judiciously. Yogic practices are also very useful to get perfect health and fitness and thereby improving the performance in various activities of games and sports. Finally, the goal of Yoga and human life is self-realisation. The philosopical approach of yoga is practical. It is applicable to all religions and communities. Yogic principles and their practice are the most effective, practical and universally accepted to achieve the highest goal of life *i.e.* self realisation. Therefore, Yoga is a panacea for all, not only for the persons who wish to get SALVATION but for everyone—be a student, teacher, doctor, engineer, businessman, political person, sports person, factory workers, house wife or labourer, healthy and even patients for keeping themselves healthy and active to achieve the goal of their life and enjoy a complete, perfect health and blissful life.

To discuss the above aspects of yoga, a national seminar on "Holistic Approach of Yoga for Human Resource Development" was organised under the able guidance of Vice Chancellor Shri Shiv Kumar Shrivastava and the Dean of the faculty Prof. Radha Vallabh Tripathi during 14-15 Feb., 1997 in the department of Yogic Studies Dr. Harisingh Gour University, Sagar (M.P.). It was felt that the papers presented at the seminar would be of very wide interest. It was decided to publish these in the form of a book. I am thankful to Dr. U.S. Gupta, Reader Department of Zoology and Dr. Y.S. Vagrecha, Reader Departement of Psychology for their suggestions and help in organising the Seminar and in the publication of this book. I also thank Shri Madhav Dhamecha, Aditya Publishers for publishing and bringing out the proceeding of the seminar. All possible efforts have been made to make this document as best as possible.

Yet I regret lapses of commission and omission. Thanks to the university authorities which extended U.G.C. financial assistance to organise the National Seminar and now to publish the proceedings of the seminar.

Ganesh Shankar

Contents

Part I

YOGA, HEALTH AND FAMILY WELFARE

Role of Yogic Practices in Health and Disease

B.L. Meti

Yoga, an ancient Indian system of Philosophy found to play an important role in prevention, maintenance and promotion of health. Scriptures related to yoga reveals that its practice leads to inner evolution and understanding of one's own innerself leading to total transformation in individuals consciousness (1, 2). Maharshi Patanjali explains eight steps to attain this state of consciousness (3). They are yam, niyam, asana, pranayam, pratyahar, dharan, dhyana and samadhi. Out of these, various types of asanas, pranayamas and meditations are being practised regularly by some individuals. In recent past many practitioners of Hatha yoga demonstrated the power of mind over body by controlling heart beat, staying in airtight cabin or under the earthern pit for many days (4, 5, 6) and also observed its importance in preventive and curative aspects of health (7, 8, 9). But due to the influence of alien systems of medicine, utility of yoga is slightly disrupted in recent years. In order to prove the efficacy of yoga several investigations are being carried out both in India and abroad. Its effect are being documented on cardio-respiratory, central and autonomic nervous system and many psychosomatic and behavioral disorders (10, 11, 12, 13). However, as there were no systematic studies available on physiological effects of asanas, pranayama and meditation perse in senior as well as naive individuals and their utility on mentally ill persons, investigations were carried out to understand yogic effects as well as its efficacy as a treatment.

Yoga on Healthy Subjects

A study on the effect of Yogasana practice for a period of two months on pulmonary function and respiratory efficiency showed a significant increase in dynamic pulmonary functions like forced expiratory volume, vital capacity, maximum breathing capacity and maximum expiratory flow rate. Also, respiratory embarrassment and increase in pulse rate observed immediately after breath holding at the level of 40mm Hg found decreased after two months of yoga training. This study clearly indicated the efficacy of yogic practice over respiratory and cardiovascular functions (10).

Left ventricular function studies using systemic time intervals on the stay in an individual asana for a period of two minutes revealed no significant changes in their pre-ejection isovolumetric contraction and left ventricular ejection periods. Also cardiac output changes were found to be insignificant during this time interval. This study indicated that even when a subject stays in a particular asana for sufficiently longer period does not produce any adverse effect on ventricular function of the heart (11).

Further electroencephalographic (EEG) and autonomic (electrical activity of the muscle (EMG), respiration, Galvanic skin resistance (GSR), electrical activity of the heart (EKG) and plethysmogram), evoked potentials and whole night sleep pattern investigations were carried out on the practitioners of pranayama and meditation. In all these subjects, on line analysis of EEG was done to obtain EEG power spectra before, during and after a particular yogic practice. Their behaviour was also monitored using closed circuit T.V. The pranayamas studied were Nadisuddhi, Suryabhedana, Ujjayi and Bhatrika, while the meditations were transcendental meditation (TM), Brahmakumaris Raja Yoga, Benedictine cristian contemplation, Kundalini, Sidda Samadhi Yoga and Omkar.

A significant increase in alpha, theta, delta and Beta EEG power value was observed in beginners and senior practitioners, with seizure like waves in the delta band. These subjects were using single pranayama for their practice. Also it was noted that this type of change was observed in all the subjects irrespective of the type of pranayama practiced. However these changes were more predominant in senior subjects than in the beginners. Autonomic changes like decrease in EMG amplitude, heart rate and increase in plethysmogram amplitude and G.S.R. during the breath holding phase of the pranayama were observed. This might be due to decreased sympathetic or increased parasympathetic activity (14). Middle latency N1 component of the auditory evoked potentials in senior practitioners of Kriya Yoga consisting of Ujjayi, Bhastrika, slow, medium and fast breathing showed decreased latency indicating hastened sensory processing mechanism of the nervous system (15).

EEG power values in senior practitioners of all the types of meditation did not show any significant changes, while the subjects practising T.M. showed an increased interhemispheric synchrony in theta band. Autonomic changes were found to be inconsistant in all the practitioners, indicating the meditation effects are individual based but not the technique perse (16).

Whole night sleep pattern was investigated on senior practitioners of kundalini on three nights. They showed decreased stage 3 and 4 of deep sleep and increased total REM duration while the number of REM episode were in normal range. This means that advanced meditators does not require more amount of stage 3 and stage 4 sleep, as their practice might have relaxed the brain cells more than that deep sleep.

Thus investigations carried out on healthy practitioners of yoga has indicated that there is not only functional harmony in different parts of the body but also there is activation of brain function by enabling heightened central and parasympathometric functions. Thus observation lead to conclude that yoga enables an individual to have energized brain in a serene body.

Yoga on Mentally Ill Persons

Preliminary study of sudarshan kriya yoga on healthy volunteers showed increased delta band power as well as seizure like wave pattern during and after the practice. This has lead to test its efficacy as a treatment on mentally ill dysthymic patients, usually electroconvulsive therapy (ECT) was given to them to increase brain activity to alleviate psychiatric symptoms. Investigation before yoga practice on these patients revealed an abnormal sleep pattern, with increased REM latency, decrease stage 3 and 4 of deep sleep (17). After the yoga practice for a period of three months they showed an improvement in sleep pattern, like reduction in REM onset latency and enhanced stage 3 and stage 4 of deep sleep with decreased depression scores.

Hence our study proves to show that yogic practice might lead to improve the mental as well as physiological well being by altering both central and autonomic functions.

References

1. The Hatha Yoga Pradipika, Transl. Pancham Singh, 3rd ed. Munshiram Manoharlal Publishers Pvt. Ltd., New Delhi, 1980.
2. The Gheranda Sanchita, Transl. Rai Bahadur Srisa Chandra Vasu, 3rd ed. Munshiram Monoharlal Publishers Pvt. Ltd., New Delhi, 1980.
3. Patanjali's Yoga Sutras, Transl. Ram Prasad, 3rd ed. Munshiram Manoharlal Publishers Pvt. Ltd., New Delhi, 1982.
4. Anandh, B.K. and Chhina G.S., Investigations on yogis claiming to stop their heart beat, Indian Journal of Medical Research, 49: 90-94, 1961.
5. Karmbelkar, P.V., Vinekar, S.L. and Bhole, M.V. studies on human subjects staying in an airtight box, Indian Journal of Medical Research, 56: 1282-1288, 1988.
6. Kothari, L.K., Bordia, A. and Gupta, O.P., Studies on a Yogi during an eight day confinement in a sealed underground pit, Indian Journal of Medical Research, 61: 1645-1650, 1973.
7. Udupa, K.N., Manual of Science and Philosophy of Yoga, J. Res. Ind. Med., 11: 1-105, 1976.
8. Nagarathna, R. and Nagendra, H.R., Yoga for bronchial asthama A Controlled study, Br. Med. J., 291: 1077-1079, 1985.
9. Meti, B.L. and Srinivasan, T.M. Branchial asthama–Management through practice of yogasana and pranayama, Yoga Mimamsa, 27: 40-47, 1989.
10. Meti, B.L., Rao, R.G., Harinath, B.S. and Melkote, G.S., Effects of yoga practice on pulmonary function and respiratory efficiency, J. Res. Ind. Med. and Homeo, 13: 5-12, 1978.

11. Meti, B.L. Cardiac performance during practice of yogasanas, NIMHANS Journal, 8: 153-156, 1991.
12. Williams, P., Fracis A. and Durham, R., Personality and Meditation, Percect, Motor skills, 43: 787-792, 1976.
13. Joseph, S., Sridharan, K., Patil, S.K.B., Kumari, M.L., Sehamurthy, W., Joseph, N.T. and Nayen, H.S. Study of some physiological and biochemical parameters in subjects under going yogic training, Indian Journal of Medical Research, 14: 120-124, 1981.
14. Meti, B.L., Study of Neurophysiology of pranayamas, Ph.D. thesis, Bangalore University, Bangalore 1985.
15. Meti, B.L. and Raju, T.R. Auditory middle latency evoked potentials in Kriya Yoga, Health Administration, 4: 56-58, 1993.
16. Kanchan, B.R., Neurophysiological investigations on meditation, Ph.D. thesis, Bangalore University, Bangalore, 1985.
17. Meti, B.L. Sleep pattern abnormality in dysthynic syndrome, Abstract, ANCIPS, Patna, 36, 1995.

Yoga and Health & Family Welfare

S.B. Mishra

Much has been said about yoga both in the west and east. It is unfortunate to see that this term is being used in a limited sense. Some identify it with physical poses and asan; some consider yoga a way to achieve miracles in life and develop psychic powers. But, there is more to yoga than this. It is therefore necessary to understand the true implications of yoga and what it has to offer.

A Deeper Meaning

"Yoga" is a Sanskrit term meaning union–a process of uniting oneself with what he is essentially. Every individual is a vital part of the whole universe. Just as one life sustains one's feet, hands, eyes, ears and bones, in the same way, it is possible to understand that one universal life embraces all beings. The yoga system of philosophy presents a rational process where one is intellectually enlightened regarding his inner nature. Yoga also shows the necessary disciplines one must adopt in order to enhance the process of personality integration.

When we speak of yoga here, we mean the integral spiritual movement leading to selfrealisation. Integral yoga implies an understanding of yoga in its completeness an all sided, all aspected union with the universal Self or God. A person must unite himself with God or the Absolute in every level of his personality–Reason, Emotion, Will and Action. In order to succeed in life, one must advance along all four lines in balanced and integrated manner.

A disbalanced development cannot promote success in any walk of life.

Therefore, Integral yoga presents a blend of four major yogas corresponding to the four aspects of the human personality. These are: Jnana Yoga–the yoga of wisdom that trains and renders the reason sharp and subtle. Bhakti yoga–the yoga of Devotion-cultures the feelings and brings about emotional integration in personality. Raja yoga–the yoga of meditation allows one to develop a strong will and a controlled mind. Karma Yoga–the yoga of Action unfolds one's hidden potentials while preparing his psychological being to face and confront life's day to day activities. Topics of health and family welfare would be taken in the light of integral yoga.

What is Health?

Health is the foundation of four fold purushartha *e.g.* ***Dharma, Artha, Kama,*** and ***Moksha.*** Before we dive deep into the subject it is important to have very clear definition of holistic health from yogic point of view.

"Health is the means of all the most sublime aspirations and achievements of man kind. It does not only mean to have a strong body and absence of diseases, but includes balanced mind, controlled senses, intuitive intellect and integrated ego to have perfect evolution of all important faculties (*e.g.* action, emotion, will and wisdom) of personality into the state of Self-realization."

A healthy person is not only a boon to himself, but also to his nation and world at large. Health is the foundation head of beauty, courage, tolerance, joy, power, peace, prosperity and creativity. Besides all the sufferings that unhealthy man undergoes which force him to live a cheerless life of dejection, depression, frustration, misunderstanding etc., he also pollutes the atmosphere around him with his negative thoughts and affects many more minds with his contagious melancholy.

All the evils, fear, discord, disharmony, pain and restlessness seen in an individual, family, society or nation are due to prevailing diseases in people. Therefore it is the prime duty of an individual and government to fight those investerate enemies of mankind,–the many diseases of body and mind, in order to establish peace and harmony everywhere. Diseases should be considered even more dangerous than gangsters, murderers and foreign assaults.

In order to achieve the goal of radiant health for all, we must have a synthetic approach of treating both mind and body. Because physical body is a mould prepared by mind.

Yogic Anatomy

Holistic health as stated above can not be attained unless we treat root disease (Mool vyadhi). For having a clear concept of mool vyadhi we should very precisely know the anatomy of body. Our present knowledge of human body is based up on Gray's anatomy as taught in medical colleges and is only related to physical body. A human being is not a composite of skin, muscles, blood and bones but he possesses three bodies. These are:

1. ***Physical***
2. ***Astral*** and
3. ***Causal***

For achieving goal of perfect health it is essential to render these three bodies devoid of all ailments. A brief introduction of all these bodies would help us in understanding the problem of health and diseases.

Three bodies are grouped in five sheaths-panch kosha:

1. Annamaya kosha- Food sheath
2. Pranamaya kosha- Vital sheath
3. Manomaya kosha- Mental sheath
4. Vijnanmaya kosha- Intellect sheath and
5. Ananda may kosha- Bliss sheath

Causal body is the inner most plane of man. It is the source of astral and physical body. It is exclusively experienced in deep sleep and samadhi (higher form of super consciousness). During the experience of joy or grief it is the causal body that operates. Its constituents are–Avidya (ignorance), Asmita (ego) and Jivatma (soul). Causal body and Anandamaya kosha are same.

Astral body consists of three sheaths *e.g.*–vital, mental and intellectual, consequently its ingredients are intellect, mind, senses and the vital force. Physical body consists of food sheath that gives rise to flesh, bones, blood and nerves.

Avidya or ignorance is the disease of the causal body. It is the source of all diseases of body and the mind. Due to the presence of ignorance, astral body becomes infected by greed, egoism, hatred, vanity, jealousy, wrath, selfishness, violence, insatable cravings for sense-enjoyments, various complexes and repeated experience of birth and death.

Diseases of the mind is called ***Adhi.*** Disease of the body is called ***Vyadhi.*** Avidya or ignorance causes mental disease in the form of cravings, frustration, worries, negative thoughts, egoism, greed, hatred and other impurities; and also it causes physical diseases such as cancer, tuberculosis, diabetes, cough and cold and numerous ailments that go to fill the pages of medical books. More than ninety percent of out diseases are directly related to the psychic upset of the mind.

Today modern scientists and doctors are rediscovering the connections between mind and body, and what is now called ***"Psychosomatic medicine"*** provides striking confirmation of the view held by ancient Rishis of India. It has been scientifically proved well defined group of modern ailments like peptic ulcer, colitis, hypertension, allergic skin diseases, various types of arthritis, migraine and mental disorders are frequently initiated by emotional stresses. Whenever there are disturbance in the mind, there are physical changes in the body. Any serious disturbance produces a physical disorder in the function of the autonomic nervous system which governs endocrinal system and involuntary response of body.

Pathogenesis of Diseases in Body

Only a brief account of the process of development of diseases would be given in this paper. Detail discussion will be presented in another paper *e.g.* Yoga Medicine & therapy.

We have stated earlier that moolvyadhi-root disease is Avidya-ignorance. What is this malady? It is an ironeous and deluding knowledge about oneself and this entire creation. It gives rise to five kleshas-afflictions which are the real cause of pain and miseries of all kinds. These five kleshas are:

1. ***Avidya (ignorance)***
2. ***Asmita (Egoism)***
3. ***Raga (Attachment)***
4. ***Dwesh (Hatered)*** and
5. ***Abhinivesh (Clinging to life)***

These afflictions affect the functions of causal, astral and physical bodies. Sequence of events in development of various ailments can be summarised as follows:

Presence of ignorance leads to development of panchkleshas, which influence malfunctions of mind. Mind has five important functions *e.g.* Right knowledge-praman, wrong knowledge-viparyay, imagination-vikalpa, memory-smriti and sleep-nidra. Disturbance in normal functioning of mind leads to various mental diseases that restrict the flow of Prana (vital forces) in the nadis (Astral channels) that permiate the vital body (Pranmaya kosha). These astral channels–nadis are linked to the physical nervous system, and are controller of the chemical balance in the body. When prana do not flow in harmony in the body causing disbalance in three humours *e.g.* Kaph, Pitta, and Vayu, then all the physiological activities such as respiration, circulation, metabolism, and excretion are affected. When digestion and assimilation get affected body does not get proper nourishment. Due to defective function of excretary system toxins accumulate in the blood stream. A severe disbalance sets in all systems there by disturbing its equilibrium to exposure to various diseases.

How to Acquire Ideal Health

In ultimate analysis all diseases are manifestation of mool vyadhi–avidya. However there are certain ailments that are confined to physical body or astral body. Therefore it is very important to apply many aspected approach for attaining the goal of perfect health. Physical methods must be applied for removing those ailments that are rooted in physical body (vyadhi) while removing adhi (mental ailments) and mool vyadhi (ignorance) astral and causal methods are necessary. No one sided approach is capable of providing true health and happiness.

In modern times great attention has been paid to the hatha yoga practices. There has been tendency to over emphasize the importance of the body at the expense of the mind. Many people have overlooked that the ancient scriptures of India stress from the very first moment the necessity for combining hatha yoga, the yoga of body with the Raja Yoga–the Yoga of spiritual development.

Performance of hatha yoga without state of mind and without the practice of concentration and meditation will prove less advantageous.

The absolute necessity to combine the mind and the body for spiritual development is the one great secret of yoga which is not properly understood by the modern world.

Therefore real health is brought about by the cure of adhi and vyadhi-mental as well as physical ailments. The goal of good health is the liberation of the soul, freedom from birth and death and attainment of immortality

Yoga and Family Welfare

An individual is the unit of a family. So welfare of the family is depended on individual. Health and well being of a person is directly related to the purity and evolution of his three bodies. Unless four foundations (emotion, reason, will and action) of one's personality are not perfected and fully balanced, there is no hope for living a peaceful, harmonious and exciting family life. Material possession is not a guarantee for a happy family life.

When personality of a person is evolved on basic principles of integral yoga then day by day he notices negative traits disappear. Sentiments of anger, hate and fear dissolve as the emotion in his personality shines forth with divine love, understanding and true compassion. Confusions about the world and himself fade as his reason becomes clear and sharp. His will strengthens unlocking the immense potential and powers of his mind. And his actions in daily life begin to take on new meaning with a definite purpose and direction.

In modern context in which term family welfare is being used, carries restricted meaning which is related to family planning, child and mother care. Yoga provides a safe, secured, natural and permanent solution to these problems. Side effects and long term hazardous complications of all contraceptives is a established fact, it is important to note that even today all countries are in search of a perfect and convenient method that has not yet found.

Yoga Holds the Key

Following the plan of integral one can perfect one's emotional aspect of personality by practising Bhakti yoga, reason aspect by adopting the principles of Jnana yoga, will aspect by following Raja yoga and action aspect by pursuing Karma yoga.

Welfare of a family is welfare of an individual. A person with healthy body, disciplined mind, controlled senses and highly evolved ego can be an ideal house holder. This type of personality is not developed in one day. It requires continuous training and discipline that starts from prenatal stage. In fact a child begins to learn even before it is born. All the thoughts that enter the mind of the mother while the child is still growing within her, impinge upon the mind of the child. So Hindu scriptures have given great insight into this prenatal state of education. It has been proved by scientists too.

Discipline is the First Step

Various types of discords and disharmony which are prevalent in modern families are due to negligence of yogic way of living and thinking. Ancient plan of living first 25 years as a student ***(Brhamacharya ashram)***, next 25 years as a house holder

(Grihasthashram), then ***Vanprastha*** and ***Sanyasashram***, even today holds the solution of most of the problems faced by present by families. Time allotted for the different ashramas may be adjusted to suit the present situation.

In a wider sense, brahmacharya ashram is an opportunity to adopt a plan of total disciplining of the body, mind and senses for receiving education, and moving towards the final goal of selfrealisation. In this stage of life young people are asked to avoid sexual intimacy and keep their minds away from things that awaken passion, they are led to understand that there is a profound responsibility involved in handling one's sex life and that if that responsibility is not properly understood one's whole life can be wasted. Adopting this principle will automatically control population explosion to the great extent.

A Great Responsibility

If one is not disciplined at an early age, he may later falls prey to numerous evils such as bad association drugs, drinking, and manifold perversions of the modern materialistic society. Life then becomes a curse and that person robs family its due share of peace, prosperity and happiness. Such a man can never become a good householder.

Householders have a great responsibility. They are the backbone of society. The Whole social structure depends upon householders. A good family can only bring forth talented children who contribute in the field of spirituality, science, arts, literature, and all forms of higher culture. One should keep the goal of Self realisation as the central theme and purpose of his life. Then only there will evolve the best type of harmony and love in the family. However, if this goal is not kept in view, love will degenerate into delusion and family life instead of promoting freedom becomes a source of misery and bondage.

In yogic way of thinking bhoga–sense pleasure is not the goal of life. It has a divine purpose. Yoga provides that insight which enables us to use sense pleasure as a mean to discover spiritual union between husband and wife, parents and children and other relationship. When pleasure is not held as the highest attainment in life, it becomes easy for a person to make the deeper adjustments that are necessary for harmonized family life. Goal of life is yoga (union) not bhoga. Once this idea is firmly inculcated in mind in early age then many problems related to family welfare is automatically solved to a great extent.

Ideally a couple should have one or two children and bring them up to become a good citizen. After that they should adopt complete continence. For the majority of people the absence of sexual relationship may seem an end of their marital joy. But this is not so. Rather, when a relationship is based upon passion, it is shallow, insecure, and fleeting. As a deeper union is established between husband and wife, there opens up a new dimension of joy as they assist each other in their spiritual growth.

Living in a Larger Family

As time passes by one should be prepared to transcend one's family, and wholly devoted to the good of humanity considering it to be his own. In modern times, the ideal of vanaprastha ashram may be practised without renouncing the family. One may prepare oneself in such a way that, after retiring he is able to share his knowledge and experience with the young, growing children of locality thus making his life as well as theirs richer and more meaningful.

If such a modern approach to vanprastha are adopted, the minds of the elderly would continue to be a joy of himself and to society. Instead of being scored and ridiculed, the elderly would be received with great honour and love.

Living with Complete Detachment

With the passage of time, one may development intense vairagya towards the transient pleasures of the senses. Then, he may seek to be formally initiated into sanyasa or one may become a sanyasi mentally and continue to perform his duties towards the good of all. Both ideals have been adopted in India. The actual goal is mental sanyasa: a mind that comprehends that "I am one with God. Nothing belongs to me. All this is Brahman".

The Ideal Family

The ideal family is like a spring garden. One can sense the atmosphere of harmony and joy just by entering in the house. According to the scriptures as ideal family is blessed with the following.

Asha (optimism): Every body's face is full of hope for a joyous future. There is hope towards the unknown and unexpected. There is a sense of joy with relation to the future due to firm faith in divine plan.

Pratiksha (waiting with patience): All members of an ideal family after performing their duty with sense of detachment wait and watch with a deep inner conviction that success is bound to come.

Sangat (good company): Good friends and well-wishers are automatically drawn. Spiritual gatherings and study of scriptures become common habit of all family members.

Sukarma (righteous actions): Every one is taught to amass the wealth of meritorious deeds.

Dana (charity): Members of an ideal family share their wealth, knowledge, talents for the good of others. Charity does not depends on material wealth. One can bring the light of hope where there is the darkness and despair. One can infusc patience and courage in others. Dissemination of knowledge is the highest form of charity.

Atitthya (hospitality): Guest is considered God in an ideal family.

All these qualities can be infused in all families of only by adopting yogic way of life. It will take care of each and every member of the family. In this way living together all the family members reciprocate in a process leading to the attainment of four purposes of life: dharma,-ethical perfection, artha-material prosperity, kamajoyous family life and moksha-liberation e.g. release from adhi and vyadhi.

Yoga and Health

Ramavatar Sharma & M. Shukla

Good health is man's priceless treasure. If one does not possess good health, one can not enjoy success, prosperity and other comforts of life. Health, happiness and peace of mind are those assets and treasures that can not be purchased.

Health is a fundamental right of an individual and is considered as a state of physical, mental, social and spiritual well being. Both internal and external cleanliness of the body are of great importance if good health is to be achieved. This can be easily attained by practice of Yoga which lays great emphasis on purification of internal and external organs, breathing (pranayam) exercises, art of eating, relaxation methods and different Yogasans for preventing diseases and promoting health. It is now recognised that for good health there should be stability of nervous system which is easily attained by Yoga which practices through neuromuscular motility and promote internal rather than external health and develop the mental, moral and psychic potentiality of an individual.

Man can live longer and can derive maximum benefit from being in a state of good health. Modern world is indebted to Ancient India for its precious gift of idealogy and technology of Yoga. The seeds of the Yoga System may be discovered in the Vedic Samhita because the Veda are foundations of Indian Culture, Philosophy and religion.

What is Yoga? The word yoga is derived from Sanskrit root Yuzir meaning to yoke or 'Union' or to join, yoga or union is the merging of individual soul with the cosmic or universal soul. The ultimate goal of yoga is the restoration of absolute peace. Yoga is control of mind and senses equanimity and seranity. It is not a religion but a spiritual methodology for a happy and healthier life.

'Hatha Yoga' is the most popular form of Yoga for its role on insistence of health. The word 'HATHA' is derived from ancient Sanskrit words 'ha' and 'tha' meaning sun' and moon. The symbols like sun and moon are applied to various function of physical and mental organisms particularly to respiration and nervous system. In Hatha Yoga Asans occupy an important place. They aim at promoting of health and efficiency of vital internal organs. Asans keep the spine, nerves, muscles and glands in healthy condition and give strength and vigour to the whole body.

The main objective of there asanas are resistance to disease, regular functioning of digestive and excreting system, a pure and adequate blood supply, a healthy heart, active nerves, mental equanimity and a cheerful and happy mind. All diseases and malfunctioning of various organs are the result of different kinds of impurities. The main role of Hatha Yoga is purification. If blood is impure, brain and nerves cannot function properly. There are six main purification practices like Dhauti, removal of bile and other stomach impurities Basti (cleaning of lower intestines) Neti (Nasal cleaning) Trataka (Gazing) Bandha and Nauli (Abdominal contraction) and Kapalabhata (Diaphragmatic breathing). But these practices can be harmful if they are not done in a proper way or not done under the supervision of a yoga expert.

Hatha yoga is the only ideal system for attaining proper and harmonious development of body, mind and soul. Patanjali, the father of Yoga stated that harmonious development of body, mind and soul can be obtained through eight limbs of Yoga: Yama, Niyama, Asanas, Pranayam, Pratyahar, Dharna, Dhyana and Samadhi. 'Hatha Yoga emphasises natural and normal method of living. It encourages natural methods and is the system of body purification leading to Raja Yoga.

Yoga alone, can give an individual a relaxed way of living. For example, a proper breathing and relaxation result in good and sound sleep. A restful mind is a key to good health. The three popular parts of Yoga are Jyana Yoga (of knowledge) Bhakti Yoga (of devotion) and Karma Yoga (of work or action). The branch known as Raja Yoga is closely related to Jyana Yoga and implies science of concentration. Bhakti yoga is the most popular yoga in India practiced through a number of temples, Ashrams, club etc. where Bhajans, Kirtans, Jagran are performed in the praise of duty. Karma Yoga relates to philosophy of Karma and means work, and action. Whatever, system one may choose, the ultimate goal is self realisation and attainment of well being.

By using different types of yoga and practicing the asanas and Kriyas prescribed there in one can not only remain healthy and cheerful but can also get rid of number of diseases, some of them chronic.

A number of diseases can be cured by regular practice of yogic Kriyas and Asanas. However, it is difficult to discuss each and every disease entity in the scope of this article. Broadly speaking, following diseases can be cured or a combination of yoga and medicines can help a great majority of patients suffering from these disorders. They are:

1. Prevention of heart attack (myocardial infraction)
2. Cerebrovascular accident or stroke
3. Blood pressure (hypertension)
4. Diabetes
5. Cervical spondylosis
6. Urinary disorders
7. Backache
8. Enhancement of immune system
9. Bronchial asthma
10. Stress
11. Gastrointestinal disorders (constepation)
12. Menstrual disorders

1. Yoga and Heart Attack

Heart disease is a great problem in our society. It signifies that heart muscle is deprived of an adequate and sufficient supply of oxygen. When this happens, heart, fails to function efficiently. This phenomenon occurs by a process of coronary vasospasm. This is a state of spasm occurring in the muscular wall of coronary retries and is caused by emotional and psychic tensions and stresses relayed from hypothalamus to the coronary arterial bed via nerves of sympathetic nervous system.

It is now established that coronary spasm is a readily reversible process. Cardiac relief occurs when coronary vasospasm is released by yogic practices which activate the parasympathetic nerves and inhibit the hypothatamic stress pathways in the brain.

Yoga is the first and foremost practice in heart disease. It gives cardiac sufferers the confidence and will.

Various asans which help in preventing heart attack are:

Bhujangasana, Shavasana, Narishodhan Pranayam.

2. Yoga and Stoke

One of the most devastating condition in medicine is cerebrovascular accident or stroke. One of the blood vessel in the brain bursts or blocked by a blood clot and a part of brain is destroyed. A normal person is changed to one who has lost consciousness vision, speech, movements of limbs, bladder, bowels etc. Yogic exercises help these victims to come back in normal life stream using asanas like pawan muktasana, shakti bandhas and gentle pranayam and can be made to lead a normal life.

3 & 4. Blood Pressure and Diabetes

These are two crippling condition which have affected millions of people the world over. Both conditions if not treated in time leads to crippling effects on health affecting target organs like brain, eyes, heart and kidneys. Yogic kriyas and Asanas help controlling these conditions and often the dose of medicines used in controlling these conditions is reduced. The blood pressure, both systolic and diastolic can be appreciably brought down to normal levels by regular practice of yoga. Various asanas which help controlling blood pressure are:

Shavasna, Padamasna, Narishodhan pranayam and dhyana and for Diabetes are–Sarvangasan, Bhujangasana, Paschimottan shalbhasana, Ardhmatsandraasana, Bhastrika pranayam.

5. Cervical Spondyosis

It is a condition of growth of upper cervical bones resulting in decreased blood supply to brain and causes headache, pain in shoulder and pain on movement of neck. Allopathic medicines afford little relief except of temporary alleviation of pain. Sometimes a neck collar or traction is necessary which is not acceptable to most of the patients for a life long treatment.

Yogic exercises keep these unfortunate victims in getting their symptoms relieved and prevent further deterioration of condition. Different Yogic exercises which help in cervical spondylosis are:

Bhujangasana, neck and solderexerce (Skandh chalan) twisting of spine exercise, chakrasna, Dhanurasna ustrasana.

6. Urinary Disorders

Symptoms of urinary incontinence, excessive urination, urethral discharge and pain an urination are common complaints of many individuals. The underlying cause is deficiency of vital energy. This energy or pran Shakti becomes depleted over many years until urinary and reproductive systems no longer possess the capacity to resist infection by micro-organism which are part of normal bacterial flora of every human body.

Yogic management of urinary tract infection is aimed at restoring the depleted energy in the urinary and reproductive systems. Surya namaskar, pranayam, shatkriyas, various Mudras and bandhas, Paschimottanasan halasan, vajrasana, bhujangasana trikonasan are some of the kriyas which are helpful in restoring normal urinary functions.

7. Backache

Backache is one of the most common disorders in our society. There is no permanent cure in modern medicine for this condition. Yoga offers a simple, effective and permanent cure for this trouble some condition. Most of the cases of backache are caused by muscular insufficiency and inadequate flexibility of muscles and tendohs. Bed rest, massage, heat, relaxation help a large majority of patients in getting relief from Backache. Different yoga asanas like Shalabhasana, ushtrasana, makarasana surpasana, bhujangasana. Shavasana help in relieving backache and restoring pranic energy.

8. Enchancement of Immune System

It has been observed that during yoga nidra healthy people can increase the number of specialised white blood cells which are responsible for manufacturing of disease fighting antibodies. Relaxation techniques have shown to increase efficiency of immune system and help an individual to fight infections much better and effectively.

9. Bronchial Asthama

This devastating condition is due to some allergic factor and is characterized by bouts of sneezing and cough and is often quite troublesome. The respiratory passages undergo a state of spasm making breathing difficult. Alopathic medicines in the form of drugs and inhalers are used to relieve this spasm. The patients have to take these medicines life long be which is often quite difficult. Various yogic asnas, and kriyas and like pranayam and Sarvangasna, Bhujangasana, Paschimottan, Vajarasna, Bhramari pranayam, narishodhan, shavasna, have been found to be quite useful in relieving spasm of bronchial asthma and restore proper breathing.

10. Stress

In the modern age most of us have been affected with one or the other form of strees or strain. There is mad ruah to earn money fame and status in the society. The body hardly gets any rest in these efforts.

Yogic asanas like Shavasana, Narishodhan pranayam, Bhramari, provide relaxation and mental peace and alleviate stress and strain.

11. Gastro-intestined Disorders

Now a days many people suffer from gastro-intestinal disorders such as constipation which is the root cause to many diseases. In yoga we can cure these patients from Vajrasna, Pawan-muktasna, paschimottanasna, halasna, Bhujangasna, Chakrasna, Udyanbandh Pranayam bhasticka and twisting exercise of spine cord.

12. Menstrual Disorders

These disorders are very common in ladies. We can cure these by some asnas like chakrasna, bhujangasna, halasna sarvangasna, paschimottan and twisting exercise of spine cord.

There are many other medical conditions which can also be helped by yoga. We can conclude by saying that yoga is an extremely useful tool in keeping fit and leading a useful healthy life.

Health and Happiness Through Yoga

S.P. Duggal

This presentation is divided into four sections :

1. Health and happiness of whom? Taking cue from Taittireeyopanishad five loyers of self are explained.
2. Keynote of mind-intellect in fighting disease, maintaining health and generating happiness.
3. Yoga as a means of creating harmony in all layers of self *i.e.* personality. It is emphasized that yoga without meditation is no yoga. Meditation is not merely reflecting on metophysical questions or achieving mystical heights or depths. For a layman meditation is a tool for resolving problems in life. How?
4. Health and happiness is a bye-product of being established in oneself. When should one strive for health and happiness? It is never too early to begin. Habit and life styles acquired in early life and supplemented during twenties and thirties die hard.

1.0 Self

Upanishads as well as modern psychologists recognise five components of personality.

1.1 **Annamaya:** The physical is the vehicle of subtle aspects of personality. It includes physical body and its biological branches-children and other close relations. Indirectly material comforts-food, clothes, house, conveyance, tools of communication also constitute our physical self. Relatives as well as material possessions-gadgets should be under our full command *i.e.*, should be assets to achieve life goals. But generally habits, tastes and life styles dictate preferences, choices, daily routines. As a consequence the individual lives under physical and emotional stress. Disease and premature old age are obvious corollaries of being governed by matter and material considerations. This vicious circle has to be broken. How?

1.2 **Pranamaya:** This aspect of personality is overlooked in the modern physiology-psychology. Yogic literature describes *prana* as electrical in nature and as energy responsible for all movements and vibrations at the cosmic and individual level. For the present discussion it is enough to note that breath is not prana but regulated breathing exercises prana. Deep breathing, rhythmical breathing lead to indirect regulation of mental operations including thought processes. Thus prana serves as a bridge between body and mind.

1.3 **Manomaya:** The psychical aspect of one's being is the outcome of past experiences. One is conscious of only a small fraction of the past impressions. Over ninety percent is forgotten but stays within the individual as unconscious store of unpleasant memories. All virational and many a time harmful behaviour is explained in terms of unconscious memories.

1.4 **Vijnanamaya:** Self concept. At the conscious level individual behaviour is regulated by one's view of self in relation to others. One may not formulate philosophy of life by raising philosophical questions like who am I? What is the goal of my life? But one's behaviour is guided by the way one looks at life and life goals. Confusion at this level is manifest all around us.

1.5 **Anand:** The bliss is an experience of spirit and it is more potent than what material, bodily and sensory pleasures can give a human being. One may rarely have a glimpse of bliss of deep meditation.

2.0 Key Role of Mind and Internal Instruments (Antah karana)

2.1 It is now universallv recognised that mind plays pivotal role in health management. The concept of health adopted by the World Health Organization is, "a state of complete physical, mental and social well being and not merely an absence of disease of infirmity".

2.2 R.R. Sharma has enlarged the WHO concept of health to that of "Profound health" which includes supramental health. "Supramental faculty refers to rare abilities like witnessing thought, controlling mental activities, intuition, reverie, bliss, samadhi, selfless love for all, and so on. The very fact that these abilities do exist in, and can be acquired by at least some person(s) for at least some period(s), emphasizes the existence in the human cerebral cortex, of "supramental neuronal circuits" which mediate higher functions and controlling action on the "mental circuits". The commissioning and operation of these supramental circuits, however, is inhibited by over-activity of the lower circuits in the central nervous system---------------Functionally the human CNS approximates a union of five brains; reflexive, reptilian (primitive, instinctive), emotive, mental-rational, supramental.----------------- The yoga practises indicating release of some yet unknown hormone, perhaps involve the syntheses of some new enzymes and also suggests the expression of some latent genes."

2.3 Kanwaljit and Sampoorn Singh highlight the role of mind in war against cancer and AIDs. "Inattentivity destroys the entire system of immunity and attentivity builds the immune system---------Health is restored when the relative frame of reference of the mind makes a quantum jump to a higher level of energy potential or a higher level of awareness". In other words immunity–the battle against disease is fought primarily by or in mind.

2.4 It may be presumed that freedom from disease is the first step towards happiness.

2.5 Happiness may be understood as a state of mind. This mental state is not proportional to material acquisitions or material comforts. It broadly depends on conditions of mind.

3.0 Yoga as a Means of Health and Happiness

Yoga is generally described as having eight components.

3.1 Yama: The social discipline.

3.2 Niyama: The individual discipline.

It may be emphasized that persons who lead ethical life as per the social and individual discipline, respond to relaxation techniques effectively.

3.3 Asana: The postural training corresponds to the physical. Postural training can take care of physical health. In disease, properly selected postures, diet control and techniques of nature cure may restore total health without any side effects.

3.3(1) The purpose of asana' or postural training in yoga is to be able to stay in a posture with comfort for long *i.e.*, serve as the foundation of concentration and meditation.

3.3(2) Postural training is now widely used as a primary step for concentrating on body movements and developing body awareness.

3.3(3) A balanced daily routine of postures should involve (*i.e.*, stretch and contract) the vital physiological systems.

3.3(4) With age exercises of the joints and stretching the spinal column are a must.

3.4 Pranayama: Exercise of vital energy. The minimum that one may do daily is twenty deep, slow, rhythmic breaths so that exhalation and inhalation times are equal.

3.5 Pratyahara: With drawal of senses from external stimuli *i.e.*, going in ward. Simple exercises for this purpose are given below.

3.5(1) Attending to any continuous sound like ticking of clock, classical music, sound of moving fan, etc.

3.5(2) Attending to one's respiration in a relaxed manner.

3.5(3) Attending to joints and vital centers from toe to head.

3.6 Dharna: Concentration. It may be as in 3.52 or on any part of the body which is not healthy, or any vital centre of the body or light of a candle or bulb, or syllables forming a mantra (chant) or an idea rectifying imbalance in personality.

3.7 Meditation: Prolonged concentration is meditation.

3.7(1) Shrimad Bhagwadgita (6:27) lays down that proper motives lead to happiness. Therefore the first step in meditation may be to clarify the objectives of life activities–long term as well as short term objectives–(Ishta). Focussing on the objectives of one's activities, habits, routines, may help resolve many conflicts and confusions bothering individuals.

3.7(2) Meditation may be done in any meditative posture or sitting in a chair with spine erect.

3.7(3) It may be done with open eyes using pen and note book.

3.7(4) To begin with meditation may be directed towards some immediate worry or problem. One's motive (s) i.e., Ishta should be identified and stated in a note book if possible.

3.7(5) Desire to be happy should be or may be gradually transformed into will and finally determination to be healthy and happy.

3.8 Smadhi: Blissful trance.

4.0 Health and Happiness when?

4.1 Foundation for the motive to be healthy and happy should be laid early when body secretions are more potent.

4.2 It is a good exercise to observe physical and mental characteristics of persons, who are senior by 10, 20 and 30 years. Three persons from each category would by enough. These observations and analyses may provide insight into probabilities in one's life. This insight may in turn provide incentive to avoid certain pitfalls and better organise one's life.

References

1. Sharma R.R. (1986), Scope of 'achievable health' enlarged. Ind. J. Clin, Psychol, 13-87-90.
2. Sharma R.R. (1988), The Quintune Brain and the Profound Health, Proceedings Conference Energy Medicine Around the world, Madras, 319-324.
3. Kanwal Jit and Sampooran Singh, Mind's war against cancer and AIDs, The Tribune 16.7.89 and 6.8.89 Magazine I.

Body Yoga

Meenakshi Devi Bhavanani

When I was just new-born to the Eastern concept of spirituality years back, I asked the manager of the Ashram in which I stayed for a single room so I could practise my Hatha Yoga exercises at my own early hours.

"Hatha Yoga!" he snorted. "Are you still so hung up in the physical?"

Since that time, I have often met with a similar reaction in my dealings with "spiritual" people, particularly in India. More common is the slight smile and condescending voice, the superior face with slightly tilled brows: "Oh! You practise Hatha Yoga?"

Yet, in my silent vigilance, I note that these self-same people never miss a meal Nor can they sit still for any period of time without wiggling this or that. Nor do they sit with spinal columns erect as they "meditate". They wouldn't think of walking more than a furlong, and more often than not, they are overweight, with bulges here and bulges there. They usually have the common complaints of periodic headaches, sleeplessness, constipation. Some even have asthma and diabetes.

And I wonder who amongst us is "hung-up" in the Physical!

Hatha Yoga is the most misunderstood branch of the ancient science. It is this aspect of Yoga which has become the most popular in the body-conscious West (though one hesitates to call the series of acrobatic twists practised in Western countries Yoga.) In the East, "religionists" often scoff at the physical disciplines as unnecessary to spiritual development. Thus Hatha Yoga has degenerated to mere head-standing, back bending, and acrobatics in the West, and is ignored by the East as "mundane."

Hatha Yoga can be used effectively as a tool to higher mind development and awareness, as well as provide a healthy body in which the other stages of Yoga can be experienced. The concept of "Yoga is Union as expounded by Lord Krishna–the BHAGAVADGITA is true in valid Hatha Yoga. "Ha" represents the solar or positive nervous currents of the body and "Tha" stands for the lunar or negative currents. Thus "Hatha" occurs when the lunar and solar currents of the body are in balance.

Diligent practice makes the body strong and supple, able to endure hardships and resist disease. Physical tensions which manifest in such nervous habits as nailbiting, finger-tapping, toe-tapping, head-herking, and so on are eliminated and relaxation is a natural condition. Vital energy increases and the body literally begins to "shine", radiating the beauty of well being.

"Man, know thyself" is the dietum of all great religious and philosophical systems, but few have pointed a concrete path to this end. Hatha Yoga provides such a path. The Pranayama, Asanas, Bandhas, Kriyas and Mudras not only cleanse and purge the body, evoking the powerful Shakti (energy) lying dormant in all human beings, but also, if properly understood, are a means of understanding the self, physically, mentally, and eventually, even spiritually.

Constant, aware practice of the age old techniques reveals unconscious thoughts and feelings stored in the mind, kept from awareness by the socially-conditioned censor. These hidden thoughts and feelings are often the very source of physical and mental hangups, the spiritual "wall" so many beat their heads against in vain.

Science in now coming to accept the psycho-somatic theory of medicine, that disease of the physical body can be caused by the mind. Psychologists have also found the reverse to be true: certain physical conditions can cause mental illness. The Yogis have known this for centuries. They call the principle

"Adhi-Vyadhi" or the higher governs the lower. The Christians may not realise it, but the application of "on earth as it is in heaven, as above, so below" is the same. The mind (heaven) governs the lower body (earth). If the mind determines the conditions of the body, does it not follow that the structure and working of the mind can be deduced by a study of the body?

The human race supposes "reading minds" to be a rare and occult power. If one knows how to "read bodies", it is easy to deduce the predominant thought patterns of the mind. Palmists know this. What are the lines on the palms but the endings of the nervous system? Physiognomists have made detailed studies of the relationship of certain behaviour patterns and intelligence quotients to the shapes of heads, the size of foreheads, the form of the nose and so on. Indian mothers and fathers bent on marriage for their daughters know the importance of a good "Brahmin nose"–a physical sign of nobility and high breeding. The aristocratic nose of the West has the same connotation. We all know the "common" body signs. A much-furrowed forehead indicates a personality which has "worries", or unpleasant thoughts which repeat themselves so often as to actually "dig a furrow" on the brow. Bright, clear, shining eyes signify an alert and active mind, as well as a healthy body. Doctors always check the eyes as part of their examination before making a diagnosis. "The eyes are the mirror of the soul". Clear, shining skin and luxuriant hair denote healthy gonads.

So also are, we working from the body, or the gross element, able to understand, the mind, or the subtle element, just as the wise women long ago rescued her husband from imprisonment in a high tower by tying a piece of string to a pigeon's foot and sending the pigeon to the window of his cell. To the string she tied a heavier string, and to that, an even heavier one, until her husband could pull up a rope strong enough to support his weight, and hence, escape.

If the practices of Hatha Yoga would be used as a tool for understanding the mind, however, the Asanas, Pranayama, Bandhas, Mudras and Kriyas must be done with "here and now" attention, complete awareness and consciousness. One must especially beware the deepest pitfall of them all in One's practice; allowing the Hatha Yoga to become a mere Samskara or habit performed in the same way at the same time in the same place with no consciousness. There can be no real benefit if the body is simply "put through the pieces" while the mind is wandering off to chappattis one is making, to a business deal one is concluding, to Dr. Kissinger's recent trip to Cairo or even if the mind is looking for God somewhere else than where it is. The mind (which represents the solar force in one aspect) and the body (which represents the lunar aspect) must be working together if the true Hatha Yoga is to occur. This I believe in one reason why Hatha Yoga has been disdained by so many: they associate it with a set of exercise done for a purpose–for health, for beauty, for skill, for egotistic fulfilment–as a means to an end, rather than recognizing it as an end in itself.

The first insight most people beginning Yoga attain is the existence of their own physical inertia and laziness. It takes mental form as a hundred and one excuses to avoid the daily session. This is usually the first shocking lesson as one begins his Sadhana–the utter laziness and stubborn resistance of the body. Be assured. If the body is lazy, stiff and stubborn, the mind will be even more so (As above, so below). (This is why the modern intellectual is such a ludicrous fellow. He fancies his mind to be of such power and importance, when in fact, it is more often than not, a tape recording of the thoughts of others, played over and over and over, along very rigid and unchanging lines). As the student progresses in his Hatha Yoga practice, his body loosens, opens and relaxes, and his mind follows suit: loosening, opening, relaxing, and thoughts and emotions are admitted into consciousness which heretofore were kept at bay by the stern and vigilant sword of his social "censor". This is not to suggest that one should indulge in these thoughts and feelings. Rather, their existence should be simply acknowledged. They should be allowed to float in the Chitta, or mind stuff, like logs upon a country pond. More often than not, brought to the daylight of awareness, they simply dissolve. These "hidden" thoughts and feelings are usually the cause of unconscious tension in the mind, the tension which manifests in the body as stiffness, soreness, regidity, or in extreme cases, various forms of disease.

When one becomes adept enough in the practices to do the elementary postures without pain, one can sensitize oneself to the "problem spots" in his body. Is the neck stiff? This indicates a mind which holds on to its ideas and opinion like a bulldog, a mind which resists change, and is often falsely proud. Are the upper legs, thighs and hips-stiff? This often means some sexual inhibition or limited understanding of the role of the sexual drive in life. Is arthritis beginning to cripple the hands? It corresponds to the mental equivalent of a "withholder": one who holds tight to his possessions, his love, his sympathy, his understanding, resisting the natural urge to let everything flow through oneself. Are stomach muscles weak and the "solar Plexus" not shining as bright as it should? Fears and anxieties have a strong hold on the mind. Does the body lack the strength or energy to hold the positions for long periods of time? There is a lack of Shakti (energy) and the thoughts and feelings of such a person undoubtedly have little effect in any of the aspects of his life. He is what is known as an "ineffectual" person. Is she back weak? This may indicate a lack of courage (backbone) to stand by convictions in time of stress, or one who is easily influenced by the opinions of those around him.

This is only a partial checklist, just for reference sake. There are of course, exceptions to all rules, but generalizations can be made with discrimination. There is no need to enumerate further, for the student will realize intuitively for himself the exact relationships which exist between mind patterns and corresponding body tendencies as his practice progresses.

Through the practice of Pranayama, one become vitally aware of the relationship of body, breath and mind. Breath could even be said to be the link between body and mind (breath in the sense of Prana). Yogic philosophy teaches in fact that man has five bodies, and that the physical body (Annamaya Kosha) and the mind (Manomaya Kosha) are linked by the breath (Pranayama Kosha). Breath is essential to the life of the organism. This is obvious. It also has bearing on the longevity of the body. Witness the animal world. Those animals which breathe slowly, like the tortoise, live to ripe old ages, while those animals like the mouse, rapid breathers, have short life spans. The Yogis in fact have postulated that each being is allotted a certain number of breaths for each life time, and when that quota is exhausted, the organism "expires". Breath is also strongly related to the thinking process, as one begins to realize in the serious study and practice of Pranayama. When one is relaxed, with calm mind and clear emotions, the breath is slow and steady. When the mind is agitated and emotions upset, the breath is rapid and irregular. It is so coincidence that the "common sense" advice to those who are emotionally upset for some reason or other is "take a deep breath". It is possible to control the speed of one's thinking with Pranayama, and to actually slow thought and calm emotions with specific breath techniques. The turbulent river of thought can be slowed by the physical control of breath, and hence, it can be brought more easily into awareness and consequent understanding and control.

Hatha Yoga practice brings an expanded awareness of the body in all its functions. One begins to understand in depth the body hungers: food, drink, sex, sleep. This very understanding eliminates craving (which the Buddha called the source of all human misery). Cruel disciplines, stern controls of force over the lower nature are no longer necessary. When the cravings are seen in their entirety, as physical desires having root in the mental plane, they assume their proper place and perspective and excesses or indulgences disappear.

Another phase of the growing awareness fostered by Hatha Yoga discipline is the realization of the effect of the emotions upon the body. Extreme worry and tension can settle itself in the digestive system, causing ulcers and upset stomachs. If the worry is an occasional one, the result is an occasional upset stomach. If the worry is constant, the upset stomach turns into an open sore, or a chronic ulcer. Constant fear or trepidation will race the heart, causing high blood pressure if the fear is extended over a long period of time. Even if an emotion is finally conquered after it has predominated for a long period of time the physical habit or sickness which resulted from it may be so strong that it continues even though the original cause has been removed. Hatred and its lesser tributaries (resentment, dislike, repulsion, etc.). Act as acid poisons in the body and make the system highly susceptible to all acidosis conditions–from a mild cold at one end to the most extreme case of cancer. Sorrow, melancholy, weeping, sadness affect the respiratory system, causing colds, coughs, even asthma, bronchitis, Preumonia.

Samskaras are circular (as is the Universe). One gets what one gives, no more, no less. Strength begets strength, and weakness begets weakness. Somewhere, somehow, the Karmic chain must be broken. Hatha Yoga is the tool to set us free from the vicious cycle, and release us into the ever-upward spiral of conscious evolutionary existence.

Patanjali was a wise man and put the practice of Hatha Yoga deliberately on the third and fourth steps of the eight-runged ladder (Asana and Pranayama). A baby learns to walk before it learns to jump. So also man learns to experience and understand life physically, through his body and senses, before his awareness becomes refined enough to grasp the significance of his mental modifications.

From that awareness comes control of mind stuff. From control of mind stuff comes one-pointedness and from one-pointedness comes the blessing of meditation.

Just as the wise wife saved her husband from death through her understanding of the principle of gradation, so also can we save ourselves from the death of spirit by an understanding of how the gross physical body is linked to the more subtle breath and mind stuff, affecting and being affected. The means to this end is an aware use of the Hatha Yoga techniques, the thickest rung of the rope ladder to liberation.

Yoga for Family Welfare

Sudha Sahni & Vanmala Vachani

For over thousands of years, the science and philosophy of yoga has been in practise for over all welfare of humanity. It has been proved beyond doubt especially now with the modern techniques of research and experimentation that yoga with its time tested techniques of development of human mind and body is of unparalleled benefit in not only promoting individual health but the health of the entire family as a whole.

How does the practise of yoga help in family welfare is a question not so easy to answer. It has been believed for centuries, that yoga is practised for renunciation from the world and to get away from responsibilities of the family. The emerging social trends all over the world and rapid changes in the family value system has put the proponents of yoga at tremendous responsibility to project the teaching of yoga in modern perspective and to cater to the basic and physiological needs of a modern family.

The following arguments more specifically seek to clarify the doubts in the minds of people regarding the efficacy of yoga in family welfare. There are a large number of Asanas and Pranayama which are specifically directed for practise in family welfare. To cater to the health needs of the reproductive system. It is in fact the only system of therapeutics that is most effective given the limitations of the research output of modern medicine. There is no known drug scientifically tested and proven to cure sexual importance or the other way sound to control increased sexual desire. Yoga has a number of very simple asanas to permanently cure both the problems. It goes without going into any further details that the practise of some simple yogic exercises rules out requirement of western contraceptives and any man in complete control of his sexual potency will also have control over causing unwanted pregnancies.

Some of the asanas cure wet diseases and other seminal disorders. Seminal incontinence and sexual hyper-excitability are also relieved. They have been so useful for diseases of the urethral system. The chitrakhya Nadi or Viryavaha Nadi (the carrier of semen) is directly effected, on account of which the circulation in the genital organ improves. These asanas make it possible to practice uninterrupted celibacy, and cures seminal disorders and many ailments of the anus and genitalia.

A very well known asana called Garbhasana is specifically meant for the female reproductive tract and is strongly recommended for woman having problems related to their reproductive system.

A young girl around the age of thirteen or fourteen years of age practising yoga will be free from menstrual complaints and further one have a very easy time during her prenatal and post natal periods. The obstetricians will marvel at the same with which she carries herself with during her pregnancy and child-birth requiring little or no anti-partum care. Subsequently, her regular and disease free menstrual cycles will regularly indicate to her as to which are the safe periods for sexual intercourse and thereby prevent conception.

In other words Yoga is not only a therapy on the accepted sense of term, but also a way of life. It is a comprehensive system of a better living. It is a total education of the whole personality.

The ultimate aim and goal of family welfare is the attainment of optimum physical and mental well being of the family. Similarly, the ultimate aim and goal of the yogic practice is also the same, *viz.* the attainment of the mental as well as physical well being of the individual. By introducing yoga in family welfare schemes the country will be able to save crores of rupees which are now spent on health care of the masses.

To conclude a healthy mind and body created by the practise of yoga will lead to excellence in reproductive health and thereby lead to an excellent family health both in terms of family planning and family welfare.

Role of Yoga in Long Life

Balaiah Kovuru

Introduction

> *"Cast me not off in the time of old age,*
> *for sake me not when my strength faileth"*

This is a beautiful quotation by a poet who reminds us about old age and says that no body likes to enter into the shadow of old age even though it is unavoidable for everyone. In old age flesh emanciates, bones become frail, sense organs become dim and energy fails and suffers from old age related diseases, such as B.P. astioporosis etc. He becomes a recluse, nobody to care him. Functionally active people even in old age maintain good health till death.

Holy sage Shankracharya of Kanchi, Morarji Desai (who became Prime Minister at the age of 82 years) lived for hundred years. Kartikeya, great yogi who died in 1952 lived for 300 years.

No one invites old age, if he is old, he thinks to go back to his golden youth. For incapable people old age is a curse. There are different rates of aging, depending upon hereditary, his food habits and life style.

Gerontologists all over the world are actively involved in research to find out the secret of longevity. Certainly they have explored many secrets. On the other side, the modern medicine and bio-medical scientists have made tremendous strides in conquering disease and death and in increasing average age of man. Certain benefits that Government has done to its people in immunisation, better public health measures etc., contributed to an average increase of life span from 30 years (some 200 years back) and now to 45 years and to 65 years which varies from country to country.

Slow Breathing for Long Life

Slow breathing is one of the techniques of pranayama. Our ancient Yoga Rishis had explored the field of pranic energy through breath. Pranayama (Prana means breath and Yama means to increase) means control of breath or to increase life force or life span. It is a science of breath. It is a technique to manage internal energy or energy pathways in the body so that the man's nervous system is toned up with which energy balance is maintained. Imbalance energy causes disease and decreases span of life. Pranayama can decrease metabolic rate of the body, the heart rate and breathing rate. It can increase temperature of the skin and the body and can be controlled to the advantage of man. Pranayama can induce relaxation of mind and reduce mental tension, anxiety and worries. Pranayama is all panacea for a number of ailments of physical and mental.

All the above findings increased parasympathetic activity and decreased sympathetic nervous system activity in the direction of rebalance. It means that anxiety and tension which work through the hypothalamic component of the limbic system within the brain are reduced. It has an advantageous effect on the autonomic nervous system and the endocrine system. Pranayama can direct energy from an overactive organ of a system, to that of an organ which is in need of energy or so to say which is under-active and thereby benefit the whole body.

Pranayama mainly acts on the pranic body which is responsible for the maintenance of energy within the physical body from where it affects or feeds the brain system. Through pranayama the inner components of the brain can be brought under control and regulated.

Slow and deep breathing was found to increase man's span of life. The yogic texts maintain that "to breath slowly is to prolong one's youth and life". Normally a man breathes 15 breaths per minute and 21,600 in 24 hours. Say God has given a life span of 100 years to a man, but he has given not in years, but in number of breaths. If the man's breath increases say to 30 breaths instead of 15 breaths per minute his life span decrease to 50 years. If his number of breaths decreases to seven-and-self breaths per minute, his life span doubles say to 200 years. In all the cases number of breaths are not the same, depending on breath rate per minute. Different animal's life span exists differently such as dog breathes 50 p.m. and lives 14 years. Elephant 20 p.m. and lives 100 years. Tortoise 20 p.m. and lives 400 years, man 15 p.m. and lives 120 years.

Sick and Obesy persons breathe more faster than normally healthy persons hence they live shorter.

I have found 25 to 30 breaths per minute in obesy people and 40 to 45 breaths in people before death. In the latter case breath was like galloping (like the speed of a running horse). Among human beings span of life varies from person to person depending on respiratory rate of the persons.

Another example of breath in terms of volume of air and oxygen intake–a sedentary person breathes about 18 times a minute and for every inhalation he takes in half a litre of air. Whereas a yogi slows down his breath to two per minute, but inhales four-and-half litres of air with each breath. In both cases, the quantity of air reaching the lungs per minute is the same *i.e.* 9 litres. Then the question arises as to what is the use of breathing slowly, when total volume of air remains the same. The answer is, the yogi obtains a greater quantity of Oxygen and expels more gaseous toxins, especially carbon dioxide than a lazy person who breathes superficially 18 breathes per minute. It is said that it is not the volume of air which matters, but the quantity of oxygen that is actually absorbed and assimilated by the body. Yogis believe that just as food is digested and assimilated by the digestive tract so also air is digested and assimilated by the body system for its nourishment. Hence it takes time for the process.

Time taken in and its retention and as well as the surface area that receives air is important for absorbing oxygen or prana shakti that the air contains. For example two factors work namely:

1. The surface area of contact between the air and the pulmonary membrane or alveolar wall.
2. Duration of contact. This benefit is not present in those who breathe superficially, on the other hand it involves a small part of the total alveolar surface. In the space of 1 minute, 9 litres of air will come into contact with 100 sq.m of alveolar wall instead of only 4 or 5 sq.m. In this span of time a large quantity of venous blood will absorb oxygen. This means a greater quantity of impure blood is being filtered. In shallow breathers a greater quantity of unpurified blood is sent back to the heart for its reoxigination and purification. Moreover the time factor is involved for maximum utilisation of the inhaled air.

In the same manner those who take liquids, or fruit juices must take very slowly so that their absorption capacity increases more than who takes quickly. The time lag is very important. That means if you keep the liquid in the mouth for sometime the digestive saliva adds to the liquid and helps absorption capacity.

The exchange of oxygen and carbon dioxide takes place only under certain precise conditions of intrapulmonary pressure and under definite time restrictions. The pressure of the two gases on either side of the alveolar wall will take 10 to 20 seconds for its exchange and equalisation. For this reason also the surface of diffusion is greatly increased by inhaling deeply and for retaining the inhaled air.

Some Techniques of Slow Breathing

1. Sukhapurvaka pranayama or nadi shodana pranayama without ratio involves slow breathing. It consists of single and alternate breathing and also double nostril breathing. This involves approximately two or four breaths in a minute. It controls the mind and removes tensions and worries, develops concentration leading to meditation. It increases revitalisation of the tissues and balances the energy of the body. Breath awareness is important. When consciously

done it registers its impression in the respiratory centre in the brain centre of Medula oblongata. In unconscious breath there is no deep breath involved. Unconscious breathers cannot control their senses. Instinctive mind predominates in them. Slow, deep and conscious breathing decreases number of respirations per minute and increases span of life.

Other means to slow down the breath rate are

1. If you relax your body and become aware of your breath and repeat so ham or hamso mentally.
2. If you stop thinking and worrying by adopting yogic relaxation and meditation. (If your continue to think, your breath rate will increase and your life span decrease. The thinking process affects the breath and breath affects the thinking process.)
3. By cultivating positive thinking, love, compassion, kindness etc., slow down the breath. (The negative thinking hatredness, anger, jealousy, malice etc. increases breath rate and decreases life span.
4. By doing Vibhaga Pranayama (Sectional Breathing) and also pranava pranayama.

During the time of stress and strain the requirement of oxygen to the body will be very high while its consumption decreases in stress free conditions to very low that is only one-tenth of the actual need. This is to say low deep and conscious breathing can be practised with out the use of fingers where ever you are and what ever the work or Asanas, you are doing. One should learn to breathe to the full capacity of the lungs. This is done in vibhaga Pranayama or sectional breathing which helps to increase the lung's capacity more than in normal people. In Vibhaga Pranayama lungs are divided into three parts on each side of the lungs and in total into 18 parts on all sides of the lungs. Each part can be inflated and deflated and also rejuvenated and the flow of blood to different parts of the body can be regulated by pumping mechanism of the heart. It is done through abdominal (diaphragmatic) breathing, chest (thoracic) breathing and also high breathing or shoulder complete breathing is done through the abdomen. This is good for blood pressure and heart patients. Vibhaga Pranayama is also a sort of relaxation.

Other Aspects of Slow Breathing

Slow and deep breathing increase vitality of the breather and develops body's natural resistance against infection or harmful bacteria or toxins. It also increases temperature of our respiratory system and fights colds and cold related diseases, such as Asthma etc.

When we inhale, the nostrils play the role of radiators warming up the incoming air. This air then goes into the respiratory system carrying with it enough temperature. During exhalation there is opposite effect. The air coming from the depth of the respiratory system the nostrils are warmed up. In this way the air regains its heat. When we inhale through the nose and exhale through the mouth the nose cannot regain its heat. Oral breathing weakness the body's immune system by loosing the heat and becoming cooler.

Time Factor

The speed of the breath also plays its role. It cannot warm up the inhaled air for want of time. The nose does not get warmed up enough by the inhaled air. If the breath is slower and deeper, the body will improve its internal combustion and will quickly and efficiently liberate the heat necessary to maintain the required internal temperature. This sort of internal temperature will promote to increase the span of life.

Conclusion

Every-body wants good health and long life, but nobody tries to do healthy things and create a healthy atmosphere around himself. If one wants to live a healthy life, it is imperative to adopt preventive measures by regular practice of yoga. At the same time intensive practice of 'Hathayoga (asamas etc.), are harmful to health. 'An once of prevention is better than a ton of cure". The cigarette smokers, alcohol consumers and drug addicts and those who consume excess of tea, coffee, sugar, milk, meat and fat etc., and fill the body with toxic waste will reduce their life span. Hence one should give up such bad habits. The yogic cleaning of the body (shatkarmas etc.) will wash off all the accumulated toxins in the body.

Richard Cutler says that goal of research by gerontrologists is "to live healthier long life with less disease". But one should remember that there is no short-cut for longivity by taking a sex pill or a rejuvenating pill. Unless one has a strong digestive power and tension-free mind nothing will help him. Good digestion and tension-free mind comes only from physical activity and yoga and meditation. Celibacy and moderate sex, preservation of semen will help to lead a healthy life in old age, otherwise old age will be like milk without butter, sugar cane pulp without sugar.

Greatest danger to increase life span is obesity and pot belly. Longer the belt shorter is the life. In obesy people the respiratory rate will be very high, hence they live short. Shat Karmas in yoga will combat the problems of obesity.

Be optimistic in life to lead a long life. Learn to be active, creative and feel always that you are young.

Astanga Yoga if practised sincerely is all panacea for all kinds of physical, mental and emotional problems and helps increased span of life. In Astanga Yoga, the first two limbs namely Yama and Niyama are very important. Yama ethical codes *i.e.* Ahimsa, Satya, Asteya, Brahmacharya and Aparigraha and moral codes, namely Saucha, Santosh, Thapa, Swadhyaya and Eashwarapranidhana, in total these ten principles are equal to ten commandments of Christianity.

If strictly followed it leads to human evolution, life becomes meaningful and purposeful. One should regularly practise Suryanamaskaras, Asanas, Pranayama, Kriyas, Mudras, Bhandas, relaxations and meditation.

"*Natasya roga na jara, na mrutuha/Yogagni mayamsha-riram*". If one does yoga there will be no disease, no fever, no death. They all will burn in the fire of yoga.

In the end we can conclude with the quotation of Manataigne. "The value of life lies not in the length of days, but in the use we make of them; a man may live long, yet lives very little". The one who is functionally active productive and creative even though he is old, he is regarded as young, otherwise he is old.

References

1. Yoga Journals (Bihar school of yoga).
2. Yoga Life' Yoga Rishi Dr. Swamy Gitananda.
3. Sputnik.
4. Newspapers.

Yoga for the Householder

Vimla Vagrecha

At a surface level one's involvement in the practice of Yoga and simultaneously carrying out worldly affairs seem to be at poles, apart. It appears that Yogin should not get himself involved in carrying out family responsibilities and a householder should not get himself in the realm of Yoga. However, at a deeper analysis, these are not the two opposite roles but complementary to each other. Let us see how these two can be intermingled meaningfully.

Yoga motivate us to change our personality and attitudes towards the betterment of life. If a householder can do so he is much better than a sanyasin who remains aloof from the society.

A sanyasin works for his own upliftment, but a householder Yogin not only works for himself but he also works for the upliftment of the society in which he lives. Bhagwadgita through the character of Arjun gives great emphasis and attach value upon this type of human-being. Out of millions in this world only a few adopt the practice of Yoga and also out of these, few rare people only succeed in achieving the true results. Man is bound by his instincts and attitudes which are difficult to change, if not enough efforts are done in this regard.

A householder is selfish, not only for himself but for his family members also. A Yogin is not so because he is not to bother much about himself and about the others. When a householder practices Yoga he is confronted with a life style which is not in consonance with a life style, supposed to be led by Yogin. Our problem is how best these two life styles can be fitted in one.

A householder wants a good health for his four purusarthas (Motivations) which Yoga ensure to give him. Yoga gives him good health, sound mind, joyful living and emotional equilibrium, through which a householder can perform his worldly affairs in a better way. Thus instead of contradictory, Yoga is essential for a householder to achieve his aims in life in a more harmonious way.

— Yoga is a way of life, which ensures perfect health—Physical, Mental, Moral and Spiritual.

— To achieve this end it begins with some does and dont's to practise them in our daily life.

— These are known as YAMA (Restraints) and NIYAMA (Observances). The negative and positive virtues.

— Yoga, however, believes in a graded course of training. One may start with Annuvrata and may reach up to Mahavrata. Or he may remain up to annuvrata only as is the case with most of the householders who practises Yoga in life. But practice of these restrains and observances is a continuous process and ultimately should become a way of life. These are as follows:

Yama	*Niyama*
(1) Ahimsa (Non-violence)	(1) Shouch (Purity of body)
(2) Satya (Truthfulness)	(2) Santosh (Satisfaction)
(3) Astaya (Honesty)	(3) Tapa (Endurance)
(4) Continence (Brahmacharya)	(4) Swadhyaya (Worship, Reading)
(5) Aparigraha (Non-possessiveness)	(5) Iswar parinidhan (Surrender to Almighty)

(1) Non-violence

This means not to kill anybody knowingly, whether a man or an animal, bird, insect, etc. A person who harms other living beings in deeds, thoughts, action or verbally is a violent person. But for a householder it is enough that he should not kill somebody unnecessary (except in self defence) or when he is performing his duties (a policeman or a soldier's killing is not a violence if he is performing his duties assigned to him.) To lead a life of Yoga one should be non-violent. A butcher cannto be a Yogi.

(2) Satya

This menas not to tell lie. It also means that one should not willfully manipulate the facts in a way which represents the reality in a distorted way and harms other. To speak truth has a great value in one's life and all religion and social code of conducts give emphasis upon it. Our formal education also emphasises on this fact.

(3) Astaya

This means not stealing but in a broader sense it means that we should not misappropriate the things which belongs to others. Thus, destroying the public property is also a form of misappropriation, in which we should not get involved ourselves. So is the violeting certain laws willfully and knowingly for the comfort and benefit of ourselves.

(4) Brahmacharya

Classical meaning of it is abstinence from sexual intercourse whether by action, word or thought with all living beings. However, it gave rise to a variety of misconceptions including that a married life is not particularly suitable for the practice of Yoga. However, the interpretation of a scientific Yoga of a continent life is rather exceptionally broad and elastic, and for all practical purposes, consists mainly of a dispassionate attitude towards sexual matters and of purity in sex, through hygienic and rational adjustments in the married life.

(5) Aparigraha

This means non-possession. However, in modern times without possessing things essential for a respectable life is non-practical. Thus, scientifically it means developing an attitude of non-attachment toward things and people and also setting a limit beyond which one will not possess materialistic things of life according to one's own life pattern.

NIYAMA

(1) Souch—Purity of body

First pre-requisite for any higher Yogic exercise is to keep one's physique and body in a healthy state. Daily routine like elimination, bathing etc. are essential to be regulative one. One should wake up early in the morning before sun rise. Clean and loose clothes are beneficial and comfortable.

The purity of internal organs are equally essential one. Throat, nose, eyes, ear and mouth should be cleaned, the air passage should be cleaned. There are kriyas through which one can clean these passages. There should not be chronic constipation and if there is any such trouble one should resort to kriyas through which bowl movements can be regulated. The food should be SATVIK and not too less and not too much.

(2) Santosh

Satisfaction with one's own life is very much needed. This does not mean that one should be contended one and should not aspire to achieve more or to do extra efforts to achieve something more. It only means that within one's own capacity and according to one's own abilities one must try to achieve according to set goals. But one should not remain dissatisfied after doing right efforts and one should not remain in a state of constant comparison. As tension is the root cause of many diseases in the modern era, one must try to keep away tension as far as possible and there should not be any place of jealousy in one's own life. A joy should be there after efforts are over.

(3) Tapa

For a higher Yogic life some sort of deprivation of body needs or endurance to difficult situation is essential. In classic Hath Yoga it has gone to the extreme form by torturing oneself. However, for our purpose mild forms of Tapa in the shape of normal fast, cultivating habits and conditioning body to endure difficult situations and building some resistence against difficulties are normal ways and desirable.

(4) Swadhyaya

It means studying self, introspection and disciplining oneself. One should set some aims of life and should practise accordingly to achieve these goals. Naturally, one should take account of it every day and introduce correctional measures whenever it needs or modify the course of action. For all these one should spare some moments for introspection and to be with oneself. A lot of reading of good spiritual literature will definitely help.

(5) Iswar Parinidhan

It means surrendering oneself to the Almighty. This is a stage which reaches in the last but practitioner of Yoga should inculcate the habit of it from the very beginning. It means divorcing one's own 'ego' and slowly and gradually gaining faith in the Supreme Power. Day-to-day observation also reveals that no system—natural, social, political or religious—can function effectively and in a co-ordinated manner unless there is an omnipotent figure in whom one have the complete faith. In the spiritual reign who else can be that figure except the Almighty or God and human-being by surrendering one's own 'ego' to him get relief from many sorrows and pains of life and fastens one's own progress for higher pursuits.

Therefore, Yoga for householder is more essential and more beneficial than it is for Yogin itself.

Bibliography

Shri Yogendra (1975) Facts About Yoga. Bombay : The Yoga Institute.

योग, स्वास्थ्य एवम् परिवार कल्याण

मंजु तिवारी

मानव सृष्टि के प्रारंभिक काल से ही सुख व शांति की तलाश करता रहा है। हमारे वेद, उपनिषद, गीता, दर्शन, धर्म सभी इसी तलाश की उपज हैं। इतना ही नहीं स्वयं ईश्वर ने भी समय-समय पर सुख व शांति की स्थापना के लिये शरीर धारण कर मानव का मार्ग प्रशस्त किया। इस अमूल्य संपदा के बावजूद आज भी मानव इसी मुकाम पर इसी तलाश के लियें खड़ा है। इस भागम-भाग में, इस तनाव पूर्ण जीवन शैली में वेद उपनिषद उसके लिये सिर्फ प्राचीन धरोहर है। गीता एवं धर्म ग्रंथ स्वाध्याय के लिये नहीं आदर्श के लिये हैं। उसी प्रकार दर्शनों के गूढ़ अर्थ केवल बौद्धिक तर्क का विषय बन गया है। फिर भी यह मान्यता है कि मनुष्य मूल रूप में आध्यात्मिक ही है। अत: मनुष्य भी अपने मूल की ओर आकर्षित हो रहा है। विश्व की मौलिक उपलब्धियों वैज्ञानिक खोजों की चकाचौंध से विमुख होकर आध्यात्म की ओर मुड़ रहा है। वैसे तो अनेक सशक्त मार्ग हैं, परन्तु 20वीं सदी के अंतिम चरण में योग के प्रति जागरूकता उसकी महत्ता का द्योतक है क्योंकि योग व्यावहारिक होने के साथ-साथ हर वर्ग, हर आयु के लोगों के लिये उपयोगी भी है। स्वामी कुवलयानंद जी के शब्दों में: "Yoga has a complete message for Humanity. It has message for the human body. It has message for the human mind and its has also a message for the human soul."

योग एक प्राचीन विद्या है जो मनुष्य को शरीर, चित्त व आत्मा में विभाजित न करके उसे पूर्ण इकाई के रूप में विचार का विषय बनाता है। योग शब्द की उत्पत्ति युज धातु से हुई है जिसका अर्थ है ''समाधि''। यौगिक अभ्यास में ''समाधि'' साध्य के अर्थ में जहाँ पूर्ण चैतन्य अवस्था की ओर इंगित करता है, या वह अवस्था जहाँ मस्तिष्क अपनी उच्चतम नियंत्रण शक्ति या सूक्ष्मतम

ग्रहण क्षमता को प्राप्त होता है। वहीं साधन के अर्थ में ''समाधि'' ''समाकलन'' का निर्देश करता है। शारीरिक, मानसिक, सामाजिक, बौद्धिक, भावनात्मक, आध्यात्मिक सभी स्तर पर समाकलन। दूसरे शब्दों में संतुलित व्यवहार एवं स्थिर व्यक्तित्व ही योग का उद्देश्य है।

आमतौर पर व्यक्तित्व का अर्थ शारीरिक सौष्ठव से लिया जाता है। पर व्यक्ति सिर्फ शरीर नहीं है उसके साथ उसके विचार, भावनाएं, दृष्टिकोण, संवेदनाएं या दूसरे शब्दों में उसका सम्पूर्ण मानसिक पक्ष भी जुड़ा है। कहा भी जाता है कि ''चेहरा मानव मन का दर्पण होता है''। या उसकी जीवन शैली उसके *विचारों की परिचायक* होती है। अर्थात व्यक्तित्व के निर्माण में शरीर व मन दोनों का महत्वपूर्ण स्थान होता है। इन दोनों का संतुलन ही योग का उद्देश्य है फिर हम इसे जिस रूप में परिभाषित करें, आत्मा से परमात्मा का मिलन कहें, चाहे ''कर्मों की कुशलता'' के रूप में समझें, या चित्त वृत्ति निरोध, हम संतुलन को ही इंगित करते हैं। वह उच्चतम ''संतुलन'' जिसे मोक्ष या मुक्ति भी कहते हैं। वैचारिक स्तर पर मुक्ति, जैसे जनक–देह होते हुये भी विदेह कहलाये, कर्म करते हुये भी कर्म मुक्त रहे।

अर्थात वैचारिक स्तर पर यदि मनुष्य अपने में परिवर्तन कर ले तो न केवल वह स्वयं को तनाव रहित करेगा, बल्कि दूसरों को भी सुख व आनन्द पहुँचा सकेगा। यदि हर इकाई ''सर्वेभवन्तु सुखिनः सर्वे सन्तुनिरामयः'' की भावना से प्रेरित हो तो समस्त विश्व प्रेम और आनन्दमय हो जायेगा। इसके समाधान के लिये योग पर दृष्टि डालें तो दो मार्ग दिखाई देते हैं–एक भावना योग, दूसरा प्राण संयम योग। भावना योग के अन्तर्गत हम ज्ञान, भक्ति एवं कर्म योग को रख सकते हैं। जिसमें भावनाओं या विचारों को प्रशिक्षित करते हैं। जैसे कि ज्ञान योग में कोहम, कोहम का विचार करते सोहम को प्राप्त करना। मनावैज्ञानिक फ्रायड कहते हैं कि ''हमारी भावनाओं की तुलना में हमारी बुद्धि कमजोर है.. परन्तु इस कमजोरी की विशेषता यह है कि बुद्धि की आवाज यद्यपि क्षीण है तथापि उसकी सुनवाई होने तक वह चुप नहीं बैठती..... यह एक बात मानव के उज्जवल भविष्य की परिचायक है। अर्थात बुद्धि को जो बात मान्य होती है, वह भावना को अच्छी नहीं लगती। *फिर भी यथावकाश लगातार प्रयत्न से बुद्धि भावना को प्रशिक्षित कर सकती है।* ''बुद्धि की उसी क्षमता का प्रयोग भावना योग में किया जाता है। दूसरा मार्ग है प्राण संयम मार्ग, यह मार्ग मानव कल्याण की दृष्टि से अधिक व्यवहारिक है। ''शरीर में प्राण की विशिष्ट गति या संचार पर, हमारा विचार हमारी भावना तथा कार्य आदि निर्भर करता है'', इसी सिद्धांत पर यह

मार्ग कार्य करता है। प्राण का सामान्य अर्थ है श्वास-प्रश्वास। रूमानिया के नाक, कान विशेषज्ञ डा० रिया ने यह सिद्ध कर दिया कि बांये या दांये किसी एक नथुनों से ही श्वास प्रश्वास चलने से अनेक मनोकायिक रोग उत्पन्न होते हैं। योग की भाषा में इन बांये व दांये नथुनों को क्रमश: इड़ा व पिंगला नाड़ी कहा जाता है, इड़ा नाड़ी जहां ऋणात्मक या शीतलता का प्रतीक है वहीं पिंगला नाड़ी धनात्मक या उष्णता या प्रतीक माना जाता है इन नाड़ियों की तुलना यदि हम विद्युत धारा से करें तो देखते हैं कि जिस प्रकार धन व ऋण भारों के संतुलन से विद्युत धारा प्रवाहित होती है। उसी प्रकार इड़ा व पिंगला के प्रवाह में संतुलन से शरीर में ऊर्जा का सामंजस्य बना रहता है।

यदि शीतलता या उष्णता का सामंजस्य नहीं है तो किसी एक के कम या अधिक होने से मनोकायिक रोग उत्पन्न होते हैं। उदाहरण के लिये शीतलता की अधिकता से कफ, अपचस या अग्निमाद्यं, शिथिलता, स्त्यान, चिड़चिड़ाहट आदि को बढ़ावा मिलता है। वहीं उष्णता की अधिकता पित्त, जलन, अस्थिरता उद्वेग जैसे विकारों को जन्म देता है। ''हठ योग'' प्राण की महत्ता बताते हुए कहता है कि ''चले वाते चले चित्तं, निश्चले निश्चलं भवेत''। कितना मनोवैज्ञानिक दृष्टिकोण है, यदि श्वास प्रश्वास धीमी व शांत गति से प्रवाहित है तो चित या विचार भी स्थिर व संतुलित होंगे जैसे एकाग्रता में। यदि श्वास प्रश्वास तीव्र या असंतुलित हैं, तो चित्त भी अस्थिर एवं उत्तेजित होगा। जैसे क्रोध के समय, उत्तेजना के समय। चूंकि मानव एक संवेदनशील, भावुक प्राणी है अत: भावनाओं पर नियंत्रण उसके लिये सहज नहीं होता, योग सूत्र कहता है कि यदि हम श्वास प्रश्वास पर नियंत्रण (प्राणायाम) सीख लें तो मन शांत होगा ही भावनाएं भी वश में होने लगती हैं। विचारों को नियंत्रित कर हम स्वस्थ जीवन जी सकते हैं।

मूलत: योग स्वास्थ्य संबंधी क्रियाओं से ही संबंधित है। स्वास्थ्य का अर्थ शारीरिक रोगों से रहित'' ऐसा नहीं है, बल्कि विक्षिप्तता उद्वेग, स्त्यान, प्रमाद सभी अस्वस्थता के ही लक्षण हैं आज की चिकित्सा पद्धति भी अब शारीरिक रोगों के निदान के लिये रोगी के मनोविज्ञान का अध्ययन आवश्यक समझती है। विश्व स्वास्थ्य संगठन भी स्वास्थ्य का परिभाषित करते हुए कहता है कि: "A state of complete physical, mental and social well-being and not merely the absence of disease of infirmity."

आश्चर्य तो यह है कि आधुनिक युग जिस तथ्य पर आज गौर कर रहा है योग ने उसे कई हजारों वर्ष पहले प्रमाणित कर दिया था। योग दर्शन में क्लेश व अन्तराय जो मनोकायिक रोगों के कारण-स्वरूप हैं ''समाधि'' या संतुलन

के मार्ग में बाधक होते हैं। अतः ''समाधि'' भावना के लिये उनका तनु होना नितांत आवश्यक है। (समाधि भावनार्थः क्लेश तनुकरणार्धश्च) योग दर्शन उसके समाधान के कुछ स्वास्थ्य संबर्धनात्मक तरीके प्रस्तुत करता है। जिसमें ''शोधन'' क्रिया, योग के अंगों के अतिरिक्त आहार निवास तथा चारों ओर के सामाजिक वातावरण के प्रति पारस्परिक सहयोग संबंधी निश्चित दृष्टिकोण तथा आदतों पर विशेष बल दिया गया है, जो शरीर को आंतरिक एवं बाह्य रूप से होने वाले दुष्प्रभावों का सफलता पूर्वक *सामना करने के योग्य बनाते* हैं। योग का एक अर्थ ''सन्नहन'' भी माना जाता है। जिसका अर्थ है–'सुसज्जित होना या तैयार होना'। उसके लिये एक उदाहरण दिया जाता है कि–''एक जंगल जो कांटो से भरा है यदि किसी को उसमें से होकर गुजरना पड़े तो एक कांटे को फेंकना तब आगे बढ़ना यह मूर्खता होगी। बुद्धिमानी की बात यह होगी कि जूते की जोड़ी पहनकर अपने पैरों की रक्षा की जाये। योग वशिष्ठ में कहा गया है कि जो आदमी जूते पहनकर चलेगा उसे लगेगा कि पूरी धरती मुलायम चमड़े से ढंकी है। ''हठयोग में 'कच्छप' इसी भावना का प्रतीक है। इस ध्येय की पूर्ति ही योग का उद्देश्य है। योग शारीरिक, मानसिक दोनों पक्षों के लिए दृढ़ पृष्ठभूमि देता है। पंतजलि दर्शन सकारात्मक स्वास्थ्य के लिये चित्तप्रसादन की यह भूमिका को स्वीकार करता है। वह कहता है–मैत्री करूणामुदितो–पेक्षाणां सुख दुःख पुण्यापुण्य भावनाश्चित प्रसादनम। 1/33। अर्थात सुखी के प्रति मैत्री, दुखी के प्रति करूणा, पुण्य के प्रति आनन्द, तथा पाप के प्रति उपेक्षा या भाव रखने से चित्त प्रसादन होता है। मनोवैज्ञानिक दृष्टि से उसका बड़ा महत्व है व्यक्ति जब दूसरों के प्रति घृणा, दुराव या अहित की भावना रखता है तो इससे दूसरे का अमंगल हो या न हो स्वयं को जिस तनाव से गुजरना पड़ता है वह उसकी शांति अवश्य छीन लेता है। इसीलिये योगाभ्यास में यम–नियम को प्रथम स्थान दिया गया है। ये स्वानुशासन तथा स्वप्रशिक्षण के लिये बनाये गये हैं। यमों में मानसिक पक्ष प्रबल होते हुए भी ये सामाजिक व्यवहार को नियंत्रित करते हैं। झूठ, चोरी, व्यभिचार, लालच की रोकथाम करते हैं। वहीं नियम शौच, संतोष, तप स्वाध्याय, ईश्वर, प्रणिधान आदि व्यक्तिगत आदतों के निर्माण पर जोर देते हैं। जहां तक योग द्वारा परिवार के कल्याण का प्रश्न है, तो हम पाते हैं कि बच्चे की प्रथम पाठशाला परिवार ही होती है। माता पिता के व्यवहार, उसे संस्कार के रूप में मिलते हैं। परिवार के वैचारिक दृष्टिकोण उसके जीवन में स्पष्ट परिलक्षित होते हैं। भारतीय इतिहास में अभिमन्यु का जीवन इस बात का द्योतक है कि माता–पिता के प्रत्येक व्यवहार से गर्भस्थ शिशु भी प्रभावित होता है। उसी प्रकार जंगली जानवर के द्वारा उठाकर ले जाया गया बालक का जानवर की तरह चलना, खाना, या

अनेक दैनिक क्रियायें करने की कथा इस बात का प्रतीक है कि जिस वातावरण में बच्चे का विकास होता है उसका अनुकरण ही बच्चे में दिखाई देता है। यदि परिवार में माता-पिता सुसंस्कृत हैं, प्रकृति सात्विक है तो बच्चों में भी उन्हीं गुणों का ही विकास होगा। कहा गया है-इंसान जैसा बोता है, वैसा ही फल मिलता है। क्योंकि बच्चा तो गीली मिट्टी है, उसे जिस आकृति में ढालेंगे, वह ढल जायेगा। न केवल व्यवहार बल्कि आहार, विहार का भी विशिष्ट प्रभाव दिखाई देता है। आहार के संबंध में एक प्रसिद्ध उक्ति है- As the food, so the mind, As the mind, so the man. प्रकृति के क्रम में भी प्रायः यह देखते हैं कि सभी मांसाहारी जीव क्रोधी, हिंसक या निर्दयी होते हैं। जबकि शाकाहारी जीव अहिंसक एवं शांतिप्रिय होते हैं। पालतु जानवर जैसे कुत्ते आदि भी यदि मांस खाते हैं तो वे भी आक्रामक हो जाते हैं। हमारी संस्कृति में तो भोजन बनाते समय, खाते समय भी भावनात्मक दृष्टिकोण को महत्त्व प्रदान किया गया है। गांधी जी ने कहा भी है-''चोरी करना एक बीमारी है और इसका कारण बुरा आहार भी हो सकता है।'' इसी प्रकार गीता के 17वें अध्याय में 8 से लेकर 10 तक श्लोकों में सात्विक, राजसिक एवं तामसिक आहार तथा उनके प्रभावों का उल्लेख किया गया है। योग एवं आयुर्वेद के अनुसार-''सात्विक आहार वे हैं जो पाचक ग्रंथी के सामान्य स्त्राव से पच जाये।'' उदाहरण के लिये खट्टे-मीठे फल, हरी सब्जी, भाजी, कंद, शहद, गुड़, दूध, दही, मक्खन, दाने या बीज आदि। अर्थात ऐसे खाद्य प्रदार्थ जो शरीर में टॉक्सीन की वृद्धि न करें एवं सुपाच्य हो, सात्विक आहार के अन्तर्गत आते हैं। उसी प्रकार भोजन तभी स्वादिष्ट लगता है, जब भूख हो। अर्थात स्वाद वस्तु में नहीं भूख में होती है। इसी संदर्भ में भागवत कहता है-''भुज्जीथा मधुर प्राय काले पश्यम् हितम्-मित्तम्'' अर्थात भोज़न स्वादानुकूल व उचित समय पर खाने से वह स्वास्थ्य को अक्षुण्ण रखती है एवं लाभकारी होती है। सिर्फ कब और क्या खायें इस पर ही नहीं कितना खायें इसके लिये भी मौतिक ग्रंथ कहते हैं-''पूरयेत, अन्नेन अर्थ, तृतीय, उक्ष्केनसु वायोः संचरर्ण्याय चतुर्थ अवशेषयेत'' 1/18। अर्थात आधा हिस्सा ठोस आहार से भरें, तृतीय भाग जल के लिये व चतुर्थ भाग वायु के लिये रिक्त छोड़ें। इसी संबंध में चरणदासकृत अष्टांग योग में कहा गया है-''क्षुधा मिटे, नहीं आलस आवे'' परन्तु आज अधिकांश परिवारों में दिन भर खाते रहने की आदत, गलत खानपान एवं शारीरिक श्रम का अभाव स्पष्ट देखा जा सकता है। यही कारण है कि अपचन, गैस, मोटापा, शिथिलता, एलर्जी, कब्ज, एसिडिटी आज परिवारों की आम समस्या बन गई है। योग में आसनों, शुद्धि क्रियाओं का अभ्यास स्वस्थ रहने के लिये आवश्यक बताया गया है। आज चिकित्सा की दृष्टि से भी इनका महत्व पूर्ण स्थान है। शोधन

क्रियाओं द्वारा श्वसन मार्ग, पेट व आंत की सफाई की जाती है, जिसमें उन अंगों की कार्यक्षमता में वृद्धि तो होती ही है साथ ही वात, पित्त व कफ में सामंजस्य भी बना रहता है। क्योंकि आयुर्वेद के अनुसार ये त्रिदोष ही स्वस्थता की आधार-शिला हैं। उसका एक महत्वपूर्ण पक्ष यह भी है कि उन मार्गों की संवेदनशीलता बढ़ जाती है जो आध्यात्मिक अनुभूति में सहायक होती है। शारीरिक स्वस्थता के लिए आसनों का भी विशिष्ठ महत्व है। सिर्फ पौष्टिक आहार की स्वस्थता का आधार नहीं है, बल्कि पाचन एवं प्रचुषण शक्ति का ठीक कार्य करने के साथ-साथ मल का उत्सर्जन भी स्वस्थ रहने के लिए आवश्यक है। आसन का प्रमुख कार्य रक्त संचार को सुचारू रूप से प्रवाहित करना है। शरीर संबर्धनात्मक आसनों के अभ्यास से उत्पन्न संकुचन एवं तान के द्वारा इस कार्य को प्रभावशाली बनाया जाता है। अंग विशेष के दबाव या तान से न केवल यहां का रक्त संचार बढ़ता है बल्कि उन अंगों का प्राकृतिक मसाज भी होता है। आसनों से रीढ़ की हड्डी एवं डायफ्राम का भी उचित व्यायाम होता है जो कि Spinal Cord एवं Sympathetic Corc के स्वास्थ्य संबर्धन में सहायक होते हैं। आसनों, उड्डयान, नौली आदि के अभ्यास से न सिर्फ नाड़ी संस्थान बल्कि श्वसन, रक्त परिसंचरण, उत्सर्जन, पाचन सभी संस्थान प्रभावित होते हैं।

दूसरी तरफ ध्यान धारणात्मक आसनों में शारीरिक गतिविधियां कम होने से चयापचन की क्रिया भी मंद हो जाती है। जिससे अल्पतम कार्बन डायआक्साइड की उत्पत्ति होने के कारण हृदय व फेफड़े की गति भी मंद हो जाती है। इस प्रकार एच्छिक-अनैच्छिक क्रियाओं द्वारा मन का विचलन भी कम हो जाता है और व्यक्ति अन्तर्मुख बनता है। महर्षि पंतजलि ने भी स्पष्ट कहा है ततोद्वंन्द्वानभिघात: 2-48। तात्पर्य यह है कि आसन-शरीर व मन को स्थिर करने वाली शरीर की एक विशिष्ठ अवस्था है, जिससे हमारे मांसपेशियों तथा चैतानिक तान स्थिति में संतुलन उत्पन्न होता है। हठ प्रदीपिका में भी कहा गया है-''कुर्यान्तदासनं स्थैर्यमारोग्यं चाड्गलाधवत। 1-17 योग दर्शन अंगमेयजयत्व या शारीरिक मानसिक असंतुलन का कारण भावनोद्वीपन को मानता है। हमारे आध्यात्मिक ग्रंथ मानवीय भावनाओं को प्रशिक्षित करने में अहं भूमिका निभाते हैं वे जीवन को संमवित रखने के सैद्धान्तिक पक्ष प्रस्तुत करते हैं। योग भी उसी कार्य के लिये मार्ग प्रस्तुत करते हैं, जो कि व्यवहारिक हैं। यम नियम, आसन, प्राणायाम, प्रत्याहार (बहिरंग योग) योग के क्रियान्मक स्वरूप हैं। जिनकी परिणति क्रमश: धारण, ध्यान व समाधि है, सामान्य शब्दों में एकाग्रता एकलानता एवं एकस्व (समन्व) है इसे ही अंतरंग योग के नाम से भी जाना जाता है। आज परिवार में बढ़ते तनाव, भावनात्मक असंतुलन की रोकथाम के लिये योग ही प्रमुख आधार

है। न केवल शारीरिक स्वस्थता की दृष्टि से बल्कि भावनात्मक सामंजस्य या स्थिरता की दृष्टि से भी इसका अभ्यास परिवार कल्याण के लिये उपयोगी है। यदि हम कहें योग मानव जीवन के लिए संदेश है, जो उसे जीने की कला सिखाती है, एवं उसके सभी अंग मनुष्य के शारीरिक वैचारिक सामाजिक, आध्यात्मिक सभी पक्षों में संतुलन लाने के लिये अहं भूमिका निभाते हैं तो अतिशयोक्ति नहीं होगी।

क्योंकि बीणा से सुमधुर स्वर्गिक संगीत तभी निकलता है जब उसके सभी तार सही हों एवं बजाने वाला निपुण हो। ''व्यास जी कहते हैं-योगेन योग: ज्ञातव्य: योगात योग प्रवर्तता'' इसलिये योग को समझने के लिये योग को अपनायें।

प्राणायाम द्वारा स्वास्थ्य एवं कायिक क्षमत्व–एक शास्त्रीय विवेचन

हर्षवर्धन गोस्वामी

कौतूहल और जिज्ञासा प्राणी मात्र के सहज और स्वाभाविक गुण हैं। भारतीय संस्कृति के ऊषा काल में औतसुक्य और कौतूहल की वृत्तियों के कारण जो प्रश्न उत्पन्न हुए उनके उत्तर जानने के प्रयास में भारतीय दर्शन की विभिन्न परम्पराओं का जन्म हुआ। गहन निरीक्षण, परीक्षण, अध्ययन एवं मनन के उपरान्त जीवन के लक्ष्य निर्धारित किये गये उन्हें भारतीय वांग्मय में पुरूषार्थ चतुष्टय की संज्ञा दी गई है। धर्म, अर्थ, काम, मोक्ष ऐसे चार लक्ष्य जीवन के निर्धारित किये गये हैं। इनमें भी काम और मोक्ष मुख्य लक्ष्य हैं। कामनाओं की पूर्ति हेतु अर्थ की व्यवस्था करनी पड़ती है और मोक्ष के लिए धार्मिक होना सहायक माना गया है। प्रमुख लक्ष्य मोक्ष ही माना गया है। यही अनेक शास्त्रों के अध्ययन से परिलक्षित भी होता है। चाहे संगीत हो अथवा काम शास्त्र, ज्योतिष हो अथवा आयुर्वेद सभी का मोक्ष प्राप्ति ही लक्ष्य माना गया।

स्वास्थ्य पुरूषार्थ का मूलाधार

पुरूषार्थ चतुष्टय की प्राप्ति हेतु मानव का स्वस्थ होना अनिवार्य है क्योंकि स्वस्थ व्यक्ति ही जीवकोपार्जन हेतु श्रम कर सकता है, अर्जित धन से सांसारिक भोगों का आनन्द ले सकता है तथा शुभ कर्मों का पालन करते हुए आध्यात्मिक विकास द्वारा मोक्ष प्राप्त करने में समर्थ हो सकता है। इसीलिए आयुर्वेद में स्वास्थ्य को पुरूषार्थ–चतुष्टय (च.सू. 1/15) एवं तीन प्रमुख ऐषणाओं–प्राणेष्णा, वित्तेष्णा तथा परलोकेष्णा (च.सू. 11/3) की प्राप्ति हेतु मूलाधार स्वीकार किया गया है। स्वस्थ व्यक्ति के लक्षणों की व्याख्या उपस्थित करने से पूर्व आयुर्वेद में ''पुरुष''

की संज्ञा देकर उसकी बहुपक्षीय अवधारणा ''शरीर-इन्द्रिय-मन-आत्मा का संयोग'' का उल्लेख किया गया है (च.सू. 1)। पूर्ण स्वास्थ्य के संदर्भ में ''पुरूष'' के चारों-शारीरिक, ऐन्द्रियिक, मानसिक तथा आध्यात्मिक पक्षों को ध्यान में रखते हुए आचार्य सुश्रुत ने (सु.सू. 15/41) अत्यन्त वैज्ञानिक वर्णन किया है। महत्वपूर्ण बात यह है कि विभिन्न संस्थानों (दोष, धातु, मल, अग्निव्यापार) की सामान्य क्रिया (विकाररहित) करते रहने की अवस्था के साथ-साथ इन्द्रियों, मन तथा आत्मा के प्रसन्न रहने को अनिवार्य अंग स्वीकार किया गया है। काश्पय संहिता (खिलस्थान) में केवल मनोदैहिक स्वास्थ्य का संकेत है। चरक संहिता में (च. सू. 21/18, 19) भी शारीरिक एवं मानसिक दृष्टि से स्वास्थ्य के उपरोक्त लक्षणों के अतिरिक्त भूख-प्यास, सर्दी-गर्मी तथा व्यायाम को सह सकने को कायिक सामार्थ्य के भाव में उल्लेख किया गया है। सुश्रुत एवं चरक संहिता (च.सू. 8/6, सु.सू. 35/31-32) में सत्व-परीक्षा मानस स्वास्थ्य के स्वतंत्र विवेचन का ही प्रयास है। चरक संहिता (च.सू. 1/41) में हितायु-अहित-आयु से सामाजिक तथा सुखायु, दुःखायु, से व्यक्तिगत स्वास्थ्य की ओर स्पष्ट संकेत है। तंत्र एवं हठयोग साहित्य के अध्ययन से पता चलता है इसके विभिन्न अभ्यासों की साधना से जिन शारीरिक, मानसिक तथा आध्यात्मिक परिणामों का उल्लेख किया गया है वह व्यक्तिगत सर्वांगीण स्वास्थ्य का परिचायक है। उदाहरणतया हठयोग प्रदीपिका में (ह.प्र. 111-78) शारीरिक लाघव, दृढ़ता, स्थैर्य, कृशता आदि के साथ-साथ इन्द्रियों की प्रसन्नता (मन सहित) मानसिक स्वास्थ्य की ओर संकेत किया गया है। इसी प्रकार घेरंड संहिता (घे.स.-1/10-11) में शारीरिक शुद्धि, हठता, लाघव, दीर्घायु आदि से शारीरिक लक्षण, धीरता-स्थिरता, निरिल्पता से मानसिक स्वास्थ्य के लक्षण तथा मुक्ति से आध्यात्मिक स्वास्थ्य के लक्षण कहे गये हैं। इसी से यह अनुमान लगाया जा सकता है कि हठयोग के अभ्यासों का लक्ष्य शारीरिक तथा मानसिक स्वास्थ्य की स्थापना भी रहा है जिससे आध्यात्मिक उपलब्धि के रूप में परम स्वास्थ्य प्राप्त हो सके। ओशो रजनीश (1995) ने तो स्वा (आत्म) भाव की मौलिक सत्ता की, निज स्वरूप की अवस्था में प्रतिष्ठित (स्वरूपेअवस्थनम्) होने को ही वास्तविक स्वास्थ्य बताया है। निजता में, स्वभाव में होने का, जो तुम हो वही होने को सत्ता की दृष्टि से ही आत्मसाक्षात्कार तथा अनुभूति की दृष्टि से इसे ही आनन्द की स्थिति बताया है। यहां स्वभाव से आनन्द की ओर संकेत है तथा आनन्द की अनुभूति की अवस्था में परमस्वास्थ्य है। क्योंकि सुख हमारा स्वभाव है इसलिए मानव मन सदैव आनन्द के लिए आतुर रहता है। इस प्रकार कैवल्य, अपवर्ग अथवा मोक्ष ही स्वास्थ्य की सर्वोपरि आनन्दमयी (सुख दुःख से परे) अवस्था सिद्ध होती है। इसे स्वास्थ्य का चरमोत्कर्ष ही कहा

जा सकता है जहां वर्तमान जीवन के प्रति असंतोष एवं भविष्य में जन्म मृत्यु की आध्यात्मिक पीड़ाओं तक का अन्त हो जाता है।

विधायक स्वास्थ्य संबंधी ऐसी कितनी ही अवधारणाओं को जो भारतीय संस्कृति की अमूल्यनिधि है आज उजागर करने की आवश्यकता है। निरंतर विदेशी आक्रमणों तथा विदेशी सरकारों में हमारी संस्कृति को नष्ट करने के प्रयास किये हैं। हमने भी पाश्चात्य संस्कृति का अन्नधानुकरण करके अपनी संस्कृति को भुला दिया। जब पश्चिम ने कहा कि आत्मा जैसी कोई वस्तु नहीं है तो हमारे मनोवैज्ञानिकों ने वही मान लिया, जब उन्होंने कहा कि शरीर और मन भिन्न-भिन्न इकाई हैं तो वह भी स्वीकार कर लिया। विश्व स्वास्थ्य संगठन ने जब स्वास्थ्य को परिभाषित कर बीमारी के न होने की अवस्था को ही स्वास्थ्य बताया तो वही परिभाषा हम अपनी शिक्षा संस्थानों में पढ़ाने लगे। अब जाकर विश्व स्वास्थ्य संगठन ने शारीरिक, मानसिक, सामाजिक एवं आध्यात्मिक सौख्य को परिपूर्ण स्वास्थ्य की संज्ञा दी है। फिर भी लगता है कि पाश्चात्य देशों को अभी भी स्वास्थ्य की अवधारणाएं सुस्पष्ट नहीं हैं। अतएव भारतीय संस्कृति साहित्य का मन्थन कर उसमें निहित परिपूर्ण स्वास्थ्य संबंधी अवधारणाओं का विश्लेषण कर समग्ररूपेण व्याख्या की जाने की आवश्यकता है। जिससे उसकी प्राप्ति हेतु समुचित उपाय ढूंढ कर जनकल्याण के लिए उनका वर्तमान परिस्थितियों के परिपेक्ष में प्रचार-प्रसार किया जा सके।

प्राण स्वास्थ्य की धुरी और प्राणायाम उसकी कुंजी

प्रणायाम योग साधना का प्रमुख एवं महत्वपूर्ण अंग है। न केवल तंत्र तथा हठयोग में उसकी प्रधानता है अपितु पातंजल योग-सूत्रों के आठ अंगों में उसे चौथा स्थान दिया गया है जहां साधना की आधी यात्रा हो चुकी होती है। इतना ही नहीं प्राण, प्राणायाम तथा प्राणविद्या संबंधी अनेक विवरण विश्व के प्राचीनतम ग्रन्थों-वेदों, उपनिषदों, ब्राहणों, आरण्यकों, स्मृतियों, पुराणों आदि में भी मिलते हैं। (पुरुषार्थी, 1983, उपाध्याय, 1995)। षडदर्शन, बौद्ध एवं जैन विचारधाराओं में भी ''प्राण'' संबंधी अवधारणाओं को किसी न किसी रूप में प्रशय मिला है। विकास के इसी क्रम में तन्त्र शास्त्रों में प्राणशक्ति, नाड़ियों, कुण्डलिनी शक्ति, चक्रों आदि अवधारणाओं का जन्म हुआ। बागची, 1939, जॉनबुडरफ, 1952) नाथ, संत और सूफी साहित्य (उपाध्याय, 1965) में भी इनका उल्लेख मिलता है। इस परम्परा में गोरखनाथ आग्रणीय हैं। वे हठयोग की नींव के पत्थर हैं। परम सत्य को पाने के लिए गोरखनाथ ने विधियों की झड़ी लगा दी। वे प्राणायाम संबंधी अनेकों अवधारणाओं के आविष्कारक हैं। इनकी प्रमुख कृतियां हैं गोरख

शतक तथा सिद्ध सिद्धान्त पद्धति (कुवल्यानंद, 1958, झा सं. 1996) आगे चलकर हठयोग प्रदीपिका एवं घेरंडसंहिता में इन्हीं सिद्धांतों का विकास हुआ मालूम पड़ता है।

बीसवीं शताब्दी काल में मौलिक योग ग्रन्थों के अंग्रेजी व हिन्दी भाषा में अनेकों अनुवाद एवं टीकाएं प्रकाशित हुई हैं जिससे योगाभ्यासों के वैज्ञानिक आधारों का संकेत मिला है। उनमें कैवल्याधाम श्रीमन्माधव योग मंदिर समिति लोनावला (करम्बेलकर-पाण्योसूत्र, 1978 स्वामी कु० नंद तथा शुक्ला, गोक्षशतक, 1958, कोक जी तथा अन्य, वशिष्ठ संहिता, 1984, स्वामी दिगम्बर जी तथा झा, हठप्रदीपिका, 1980, स्वामी दिगम्बर जी एवं घरोटे, धेरंड संहिता, 1978, घरोटे तथा बेडेकर, बृहद्योगीयाज्ञवल्क्य स्मृति 1980) बिहार योग विद्यालय के (स्वामी मुक्ति बोधानंद, हठयोग प्रदीपिका 1985, स्वामी सत्यसगानंद तत्वशुद्धि, 1984, स्वामी निरंजना नंद, प्राणविद्या, 1994) तथा ओशोइन्टरनेशनल फाउन्डेशन के (चिन्मय एवं सत्यार्थी पातन्जलयोगसूत्र, 1994, स्वामी बोधि सत्व, कुंडलिनी और तंत्र 1951, बोधिसत्व कुण्डलिनी और सात शरीर 1989, बोधिसत्व कुण्डलिनी जागरण व शक्तिषात, 1995, बोधिसत्व, कुण्डलिनी यात्रा, 1991, बोधिसत्व, चेतना का सूर्य, 1990 के प्रकाशन प्रमुख हैं। वैज्ञानिक अनुसंधान की दुष्टि से कैवल्यधाम से प्रकाशित अब तक के योगमीमांसा त्रैमासिक पत्रिका के 31 अंक, बिहार योग विद्यालय के योग तथा योग विद्या की मासिक पत्रिकाएं उल्लेखनीय हैं।

प्राणायाम पर शोध की आवश्यकता एवं उसका महत्व

उपरोक्त ऐतिहासिक साहित्य में प्राण शब्द के अनेकों पर्याय, प्राण का स्थूल एव सूक्ष्म शरीर का अंग होने, प्राणों के नियमित व्यापार करते रहने से स्वास्थ्य लाभ, प्राणायाम कोश, आत्मा के साथ प्राणों का घनिष्ट संबंध, प्राणोपासना, प्राणायाम कोश की साधना पद्धति, प्राण निरोध न करने से हानि, प्राणायाम से रोग विनाश, प्राणायाम के अनेकों भेद, उनकी विधि और लाभ, प्राणायाम की तैयारी, विशेष स्थान काल भोजन की व्यवस्था आदि के जो उल्लेख मिलते हैं उनसे ही यह अनुमान लगाया जा सकता है कि प्राणायाम योग साधना का ही नहीं अपितु वर्तमान परिस्थितियों के परिवेक्ष में भी परम स्वास्थ्य का सशक्त माध्यम बनाया जा सकता है।

योग के बढ़ते प्रचार-प्रसार के कारण शोधकर्ताओं का औतुसक्य भी बढ़ा है। इसलिए प्राथमिक आवश्यकता इस बात की है कि प्राणायाम संबंधी सामग्री जो वेदों, उपनिषदों, ब्राहमणों, आरण्यकों, महाभारत, गीता, स्मृतियों, पुराणों,

पातन्जल योगसूत्र, तंत्रशास्त्र, आयुर्वेद एवं हाठयोग ग्रन्थों, स्वरशास्त्र, ज्योतिष आदि के साहित्य में अथवा जहां कहीं भी उपलब्ध होते हों उसे एकत्र किया जाये, विभिन्न पक्षों का वर्गीकरण किया जाये, विभिन्न मतों का तुलनात्मक अध्ययन किया जाये जिससे वैचारिक समानता एवं भेद का अध्ययन हो सके, तकनीकी शब्दावली की विभिन्न प्रसंगों में व्याख्या की जाये तथा उनका विकास क्रम सुनिश्चित किया जाये। अभी तक किसी भी अकेले एक योगाभ्यास पर ऐसा सुनियोजित अध्ययन नहीं किया गया है। ऐतिहासिक एवं शास्त्रीय दृष्टि से प्रस्तुत शोधकार्य योजना अत्यंत महत्वपूर्ण होने की पूरी संभावना है क्योंकि प्राणायाम के नये घटकों के उद्घाटन से तथा तुलनात्मक समालोचना से यह सामग्री वैज्ञानिक प्रयोगशालाओं में भावी अनुसंधानों को पृष्ठभूमि प्रदान कर सकेगी।

संदर्भ ग्रन्थ सूची

1. अग्निदेव, (1960): सुश्रुत संहिता, मोतीलाल बनारसीदास, वाराणसी।
2. ओशो रजनीश (1995): कुडलिनी जागरण व शक्तिपात, डायमंड पाकेट बुक्स प्रा. लि.
3. नागेन्द्र, एच.आर. (1996): प्राणायाम–कला एवं विज्ञान, विवेकानंद केन्द्र योग प्रकाशन, बंगलौर।
4. पुरुषार्थी, योगेन्द्र (1983): वेदों में योग विद्या, योगिक शोध संस्थान, योगधाम, ज्वालापुर, (हरिद्वार), 1983।
5. स्वामी दिगम्बर जी एवं झा. पीताम्बर (1980): हठप्रदीपिका, कैवल्यधाम श्रीमन् मा. यो.मं. समिति, लोनावला, पूना।
6. सिंह, विजयबहादुर (सं. 2015) प्राणायाम मीमांसा, हिन्दी साहित्य कुटीर, वाराणसी।

योग एक जीवन–पद्धति

रामेश्वर दास गुप्त

योग एक जीवन–पद्धति है। इस जीवन–पद्धति का प्रथम उद्देश्य मानव को सही अर्थ में मनुष्य बनाना है। मनुष्य तब बनता है जब उसमें मनुष्यता का प्रादुर्भाव होता है। मनुष्य बनने के लिए सर्वप्रथम यमों और नियमों का पालन करना और उन्हें जीवन में धारण करना अनिवार्य है। इससे उसकी बुद्धि जागृत होगी; उसमें विवेक और ज्ञान का उदय होगा।

यम का जहाँ तक सम्बन्ध है, वह सबसे पहले मनुष्य को अहिंसक बनाता है। जब मनुष्य अहिंसक हो जाएगा तो वह न केवल मनुष्य का, अपितु प्राणिमात्र का रक्षक बन जायेगा। वह किसी की हत्या तो करेगा ही नहीं, प्रत्युत वह मन, वचन और कर्म से किसी को कश्ट भी नहीं पहुँचाएगा और किसी को शारीरिक पीड़ा अथवा मानसिक आघात भी नहीं देगा। सामाजिक दृष्टि से वह किसी का अनादर भी नहीं करेगा।

यम का दूसरा आचारण है 'सत्य'। सत्य का अर्थ है सच बोलना और सच्चा व्यवहार करना। सत्य भगवान को भी कहते हैं। सत्य हमें भगवान के निकट ले जाता है। सत्य बोलने वाले का वचन अमोघ हो जाता है। जो व्यक्ति सत्य को अपने जीवन में (मन, वचन और कर्म में) पूरी तरह धारण कर लेगा, वह भगवान को भी जान लेगा।

यम के तीसरे चरण 'अस्तेय' कहा जहाँ तक सम्बन्ध है, इसका सीधा–सादा अर्थ है चोरी न करना। चोरी, बेईमानी, घूसखोरी, छल–कपट आदि को त्यागकर, अपनी कमाई से अपने अधिकार के जीवन–निर्वाह के साधनों से ही संतुष्ट रहना और किसी के अधिकार का अनुचित ढंग से अपहरण न करना ही अस्तेय है।

अस्तेय के पालन से मनुष्य को हीरे-जवाहरातों से बढ़कर परम शांति के रूप में सच्ची दौलत मिलती है।

यम का चौथा आचरण है 'ब्रह्मचर्य'। ब्रह्मचर्य का जहाँ तक सम्बन्ध है, इस पर बहुत कुछ लिखा जा सकता है; एक अच्छी मोटी पुस्तक भी छोटी पड़ सकती है। इस विषय में अनेक पुस्तकें हैं भी। यदि हम कुछ शब्दों में कहना चाहें तो कह सकते हैं कि गृहस्थ जीवन में रहते हुए भी संयमपूर्वक दाम्पत्य-जीवन का भोग करें। ऐसा करने से शरीर लम्बी आयु तक उत्साहयुक्त, रोगरहित, सबल और पवित्र तथा मन प्रसन्न, सबल और पवित्र रहता है।

यम का पाँचवाँ आचरण है 'अपरिग्रह'। अपरिग्रह का पालन करते हुए मनुष्य अपनी आवश्यकता से अधिक संग्रह नहीं करेगा। कबीर ने भी कहा है:

जो जल बाढ़े नाव में, घर में बाढ़े दाम।
दोऊ हाथ उलीचिये, यही सयानो काम।।

जो व्यक्ति अति संग्रह नहीं करता है, वह लोभ से भी दूर रहता है। लोभ सारे पापों की जड़ है। अतः जीवन में संग्रह की वृत्ति को पनपने नहीं देना चाहिए।

नियम का पहला आचरण है 'शौच'। बाहरी शौच का पालन करने में जल, साबुनादि से अपने शरीर, वस्त्रादि को स्वच्छ रखना, योग-विधि से जल पीकर शरीर के आन्तरिक अंगों की शुद्धि करना आदि आता है। मन को स्वच्छ रखने के लिए राग, द्वेष, घृणा, वैर, ईर्ष्या आदि दुर्भावनाओं का त्याग भी बहुत जरूरी है। तनाव अनेक रोगों का मूल कारण है। अतः मन को तनावरहित, शान्त और आनन्दित रखने के लिए मित्रता, करुणा, प्रसन्नतादि सद्भावनाओं को ग्रहण करना आन्तरिक शौच कहलाता है।

नियम का दूसरा आचरण है 'संतोष'। संतोष को धारण करने वाला संतोषी बन जाता है। वह हर हालत में आनन्दित रहता है। ठीक ही कहा गया है:

'जब आवे संतोष धन, सब धन धूरि समान'।

नियम का तीसरा आचरण है 'तप'। दैनिक जीवन में भूख-प्यास, निन्दा-स्तुति, सुख-दुख, मान-अपमान, हानि-लाभ आदि को विधि का विधान मानकर प्रसन्नता से सह लेना तथा विरोध सहकर भी दूसरों की भलाई में लगे रहना तप कहलाता है। तप करने वाला साधक धैर्यपूर्वक योगाभ्यास करता है; साधना करता है। उसमें भरपूर सहनशक्ति उत्पन्न हो जाती है। वह नीरोग, स्वस्थ, सक्रिय और सुन्दर बना रहता है, जल्दी बूढ़ा नहीं होता और उनके स्वास्थ्य और

सौन्दर्य को देखकर, उसके आसपास के लोग भी, उसके आचरण को अपनाकर सुखी रहने का प्रयत्न करते हैं।

नियम का चौथा आचरण है 'स्वाध्याय'। स्वाध्याय करने वाला व्यक्ति जहाँ श्रेष्ठ साहित्य का स्वाध्याय करता है वहाँ 'स्व' अर्थात् अपने वास्तविक स्वरूप का भी अध्ययन एवं चिंतन करता है। इससे वह परमात्मा के साक्षात्कार की ओर उन्मुख हो जाता है। उसे किसी इलाज की, किसी चिकित्सा की आवश्यकता नहीं रहती, क्योंकि अधिकतर रोगों की उत्पत्ति का कारण विचार-शक्ति का दूषित होना ही है।

नियम का पाँचवा आचरण है 'ईश्वर-प्रणिधान' इसका अर्थ है-अपने आपको ईश्वर के प्रति समर्पित करना, रात-दिन उसका जप-ध्यान करना, सब मनुष्यों को उसी की सन्तान समझकर, बिना स्वार्थ सबकी भलाई में लगे रहना तथा अपने अच्छे कर्मों से भी किसी दुनियावी फल न चाहकर, उनको भगवान की प्रसन्नता के लिए निरंतर करते चले जाना और अपने आपको पूरी तरह उसके सामने समर्पित कर देना।

जब व्यक्ति अपने आपको परमात्मा के प्रति समर्पित कर देता है, तो उसे कोई भी किसी प्रकार की चिन्ता या भय नहीं रहता। परमात्मा के प्रति समर्पण की बात तो है ही, परन्तु आज के जन--जीवन में मनुष्य यदि प्राणी-मात्र के प्रति समर्पित हो जाए तो भी काफी है; तब उसे किसी से और किसी को उससे, किसी भी प्रकार का द्वेष नहीं रहेगा। वह सामाजिक सद्भाव और प्रेम से भरपूर होकर, आनन्द से तरंगित हो उठेगा। हमारे पूर्वजों का सुझाया हुआ कर्मयोग यही है।

आसनों का जहाँ तक सम्बन्ध है, इन आसानों के अभ्यास से मांस-पेशियाँ तनावमुक्त होती हैं; जोड़ों में लचीलापन आता है; आन्तरिक अंग प्रभावित होते हैं; रक्त-संचार भली-भांति होने लगता है; शरीर नीरोग, स्वस्थ, सबल और सक्रिय बन जाता है। ध्यानात्मक आसनों के अभ्यास द्वारा मन स्थिर होता है। इन आसनों का अभ्यास करते समय सिर, गर्दन और मेरुदण्ड को सीधा रखने के साथ-साथ शरीर को ढीला रखना चाहिए।

प्राणायाम के अभ्यास से मन और प्राण का संतुलन बना रहता है, राग-द्वेषादि मनोविकार क्षीण होते हैं, मन और इन्द्रियाँ शान्त हो जाती हैं; नस, नाड़ियाँ शुद्ध और बलिष्ठ हो जाती हैं। वात, पित्तादि दोष सम रहते हैं और शरीर की सभी धातुएँ और मल ठीक कार्य करते हैं। फलतः मनुष्य नीरोग और तेजस्वी बना

रहता है। प्राणायाम से मानसिक एकाग्रता, स्मृति, संयमशक्ति तथा शान्ति प्राप्त होने के साथ–साथ आयु भी बढ़ जाती है।

प्रत्याहार के माध्यन से इन्द्रियों को अन्तर्मुखी किया जाता है। ध्यान में प्रवेश पाने के लिए इसमें आँख, नाक, कान जीभ और त्वचा आदि इन्द्रियों को बाहरी दुनिया से हटाकर, अन्तर्मुख करना होता है। इससे जहाँ मन को स्थिर तथा सबल बनाने में मदद मिलेगी, वहीं मन को सब ओर से हटाकर एक विषय में लगाने का मार्ग खुल जाएगा, उसी का नाम धारणा है। धारणा के निरन्तर अभ्यास से साधक ध्यान–मग्न हो जाता है। ध्यान द्वारा मन नीरोग, स्वस्थ और शान्त बने रह सकते हैं। ध्यान द्वारा हम अपनी छिपी हुई शक्तियों को न केवल जान सकते हैं, अपितु जगा भी सकते हैं और आगे चलकर चमत्कार भी होने लगते हैं। वे चमत्कार गोपनीय होते हैं। सच्चा साधक उन्हें किसी के सामने व्यक्त नहीं करता, प्रत्युत उनका साक्षात् प्रत्यक्ष कर सकता है। ध्यान करने के लिए साधक को किसी भी अभ्यस्त ध्यानासन जैसे–सुखासन, सिद्धासन अथवा पद्मासन में बैठकर, आँखों को कोमलता के साथ बन्द करके, अपने श्वास–प्रश्वास को देखना होता है। ध्यान उसी पर टिकाया जाता है। इस साधना के पक्का होने पर साधक अपने अन्तर में झाँकते हुए और गहरे उतरते हुए प्रकाश और आनन्द को तो प्राप्त कर ही लेता है। इसके अतिरिक्त न जाने क्या–क्या सच्ची कमाई प्राप्त कर सकता है, जो सांसारिक सम्पत्ति की तुलना में अधिक महत्त्वपूर्ण तथा सदा रहने वाली है।

आसन लगाकर दोनों हाथों की तर्जनी अंगुलियों के सिरों को दोनों कानों में डालकर, कोमलता से आँखें बन्द करके अनाहतनाद करके सुना जाता है। इससे भी मन को एकाग्र करने में सहायता मिलती है।

योग कथा का विषय है नहीं, प्रत्युत क्रियात्मक अभ्यास का विषय है। लगभग 35 वर्ष पूर्व मेरे एक मित्र राममूर्ति रेणु कुछ दिन मेरे पास रुके थे। तेलुगु–भाषी होकर भी उन्होंने बनारस हिन्दू–विश्वविद्यालय से हिन्दी में एम.ए. किया था। एक दिन वे दिल्ली विश्वविद्यालय में अपने किसी मित्र से मिलने गए। सायंकाल लौटे तो मुझसे कहा, ''भैया! मैं मिल आया। उनके घर में बैठकर ऐसा नहीं लगा कि मैं किसी भारतीय परिवार में बैठा हूँ। वहाँ तो ऐसा लग रहा था कि मैं किसी विदेशी घर में हूँ। हिन्दी के प्राध्यापक होकर भी उनके जीवन–शैली में भारतीयता नहीं है। उन्होंने तुलसी पढ़ाया तो है पर तुलसी बनाया नहीं।''

इस विश्वविद्यालय ने बहुत से छात्र–छात्राओं को योगाचार्य, डाक्टर आदि उपाधियों से विभूषित किया होगा। पर मेरे विचार में योग की उपाधियाँ देने से

अधिक महत्त्वपूर्ण एक सच्चा योगी बनाना है। अत: विश्वविद्यालयों के योग-विभागों में, योग की उच्च साधनाएँ कराने की व्यवस्था भी होनी चाहिए।

योग आत्म-साक्षात् करने, आत्मदेव के दर्शन करने, आत्मा को परमात्मा के ध्यान में लय करने तथा परमानन्द प्राप्त करने का साधन है। परन्तु अनुदान और इलाज के सहारे उसे भौतिकवाद की दृष्टि से देखा जा रहा है, जबकि मेरे विचार से योग और विज्ञान एक दूसरे के पूरक हैं; विरोधी नहीं। जहाँ आप योग को विज्ञान की कसौटी पर कसते हैं, वहाँ विज्ञान को भी तो योग की कसौटी पर कसने का प्रयास कीजिए। योग को जीवन-पद्धति न मानकर, मात्र-चिकित्सा मानने से योग एक गहन अध्यात्म-विज्ञान न रह कर मात्र-बाहरी व्यायाम तथा पूर्णत: भोग का पर्याप्य बन जायेगा। क्या आप इस खतरे को मोल लेना चाहते हैं? जहाँ आप बहिर्मुखी प्रयासों में लगे हुए हैं, वहाँ कुछ अन्दर की ओर भी तो झाँकिए; स्थूल से सूक्ष्मता की ओर बढ़िए।

हमें जो कुछ भी कार्य करना है, इस शरीर द्वारा ही करना है। कहा भी है-''शरीमाद्यं खलु धर्मसाधनम्।'' किन्तु शरीर तो वह भी है जो चिकित्सालय में लेटा हुआ है। परन्तु उस शरीर से कोई कार्य होना सम्भव नहीं है। इसके लिए नीरोग, स्वस्थ और सक्रिय शरीर की आवश्यकता है। शरीर को स्वस्थ और सक्रिय बनाए रखने के लिए हमें अपने खान-पान, रहन-सहन और आचार-विचार पर पूरा ध्यान देना होगा। साधक सात्त्विक भोजन करें, अखाद्य का भक्षण नहीं करें, समय पर खाएं, हर समय चरते नहीं रहें, जल्दी सोएँ, जल्दी उठें, किसी का बुरा न चाहें, किसी से द्वेष नहीं करें, राग की प्रवृत्ति से भी दूर रहें और यम-नियम का पालन करते हुए निरन्तर साधना करते रहें।

इस जीवन-पद्धति से मैं यह तो नहीं कह सकता कि समाज के सभी रोगों का शमन हो जाएगा परन्तु इतना अवश्य कह सकता हूँ कि जिस दिन, जिस समय भी समाज के लोगों ने योग को अपने जीवन में अपना लिया, उसी समय से वे अपने अन्दर जो कमियाँ महसूस करते हैं, वे आगे नहीं बढ़ पायेंगी। एक दिन ऐसा भी आयेगा कि वे कमियाँ अपने आप दूर हो जायेंगी, धुल जायेंगी, साधकों के शरीर और अंत:करण कुन्दन के समान शुद्ध और गंगाजल के समान पवित्र हो जाऐंगें तथा वे सदा आनन्दित रहेंगे। फिर बीमारियों का उनके निकट आने का प्रश्न ही नहीं उठेगा। जब मनुष्य नीरोग, स्वस्थ, सबल, सक्रिय और प्रसन्न रहेंगे तो यौगिक चिकित्सा की या प्राकृतिक चिकित्सा की अथवा अन्य किसी चिकित्या-पद्धति के चिकित्सालयों की क्या आवश्यकता रह जायेगी? फिर जो समय और सम्पत्ति इन पर बरबाद हो रहे हैं, उस समय और उस सम्पत्ति

को समाज के निर्माण और राष्ट्र की उन्नति के लिए लगाया जा सकेगा, जिससे समाज, संस्कृति तथा राष्ट्र का कल्याण होगा। अतः मेरे विचार से योग को एक आदर्श जीवन–पद्धति के रूप में अपनाकर समग्र राष्ट्र के जीवन में उतारना नितांत आवश्यक है।

ओउम् शान्तिः शान्तिः शान्तिः

YOGA, MEDICINE AND THERAPY

Yoga, Medicine and Therapy

S.B. Mishra

Along with material advancement and economic development there is massive increase in various types of ailments through out world. No country can claim itself to be free of diseases. Every day new health problems and new diseases with complex aetiology and unknown causes are reported.

Inspite of best possible precautions and remedies adopted, we see many diseases thought to be eradicated, crop up again more vehemently. Due to rapid communication and interaction between people no country is safe. If an epidemic breaks out in any part of the globe it will soon spread in all countries.

It has been proved beyond doubts that there is no system that can be called safe, secured, effective and universally accepted for the treatment of various ailments. Modern medical scientists have started realizing the limitations of symptomatic treatment. Because they are now convinced that root of all diseases may not be in physical body. A subtle link between mind and body has been established scientifically. Now "**psychosomatic disorder**" is an important chapter in medical curriculum.

Yoga as a Therapy

Inspite of recent advancement in various fields of medical science, entire world is looking for an alternative mode of treatment. Yoga is considered as the future hope and the only light in darkness.

Although diseases can be cured by yoga but great yogis, sages and expounders of yoga never advocated to use yoga as a pathy for curing diseases. They looked disease from a different angle. Yoga recognises only one disease that is **Mool vyadhi-Avidya** (ignorance). All other ailments are only a ramifications of the mool vyadhi. Once this root cause is eradicated one can enjoy perfect health and happiness without being affected by any disease. Yoga may be called a pathy in that border sense. It prescribes various remedies for breaking the fetters of avidya the root disease.

Limited Approach

For the last few decades yoga is being prescribed as an alternative method of treatment. Desperate people through out world are running towards so called yoga clinic with a great expectation. But what is the real picture? Are people getting relief? Is yoga effective in removing various illness? As a alopathic doctor I come across many patients who have reported that they did try and taken various courses of yoga treatment with no result. Then one may ask "Is yoga ineffective as an alternative mode of treatment?" No. Basic cause of failure is different. So called yoga charyas and yoga therapists are themself ignorant about deep understanding of yogic science of cure.

There is over emphasis on physical form of yoga completely ignoring its deeper and more profound aspects. Presently people are prescribing certain asans and kriyas for certain diseases. Patients go on practising these asans for some time and when they do not find any relief, discontinue their practice with a wrong notion that yoga too has failed in giving desired result. This is what exactly going on presently.

Curing a disease is not so simple. One can't hope to get good flowers and fruits by irrigating leaves and branches. One has to look after the roots. Once total implication of yoga is understood it can be utilised to get cure of all types of ailments. Diseases affect personality. So it is important to under stand human personality in its entirety before going deep into therapeutic aspect of yoga.

Four Foundations of Human Personality

A person is not made of only material constituents that go to form skin, muscles, blood and bone as basic ingredients of its physical body. Rather, entire human personality is constituted of two basic factors:

1. Matter (jada)
2. Consciousness (chetana)

These two basic ingredients give rise to four foundations of human personality:

1. Action
2. Emotion
3. Will and
4. Wisdom

A human being expresses himself in these four dimentions. Although these are classified as independent groups but one contains some percentage of rest of the three *e.g.* when action aspect is being expressed there is some amount of emotion, will as well as wisdom underlying it. In an ideal personality these four are developed in its fullness. It is important to note that there is two ways communication. These four factors have emerged from combination of matter and consciousness, there by influenced by them. On the other hand, these factors influence basic originating cause *e.g.* matter and consciousness. Keeping all these points in view now is the time to know what really yoga is. Because edifice of yogic medicine and therapy rests on correct understanding of yoga.

What is Yoga

"Yoga" is a Sanskrit term meaning union—a process of uniting oneself with what he is essentially. Every individual is a vital part of the whole universe. Just as one life sustains one's feet, hands, eyes, ears and bones, in the same way, it is possible to understand that one universal life embraces all beings. The yoga system of philosophy presents a rational process where one is intellectually enlightened regarding his inner nature. Yoga also shows the necessary disciplines one must adopt in order to enhance the process of personality integration.

When we speak of yoga here, we mean the integral spiritual movement leading to self-realization. Integral yoga implies an understanding of yoga in its completeness an all sided, all aspected union with the universal Self or God. A person must unite himself with God or the Absolute in every level of his personality–**Reason, Emotion, Will** and **Action.** In order to succeed in life, one must advance along all four lines in balanced and integrated manner. A disbalanced development cannot promote success in any walk of life.

Therefore, Integral yoga presents a blend of four major yogas corresponding to the four aspects of the human personality. These are: **Jnana Yoga**–the yoga of wisdom that trains and renders the reason sharp and subtle. **Bhakti yoga**–the yoga of Devotion-cultures the feelings and brings about emotional integration in the personality. **Raja yoga**–the yoga of meditation allows one to develop a strong will and a controlled mind. **Karma yoga**–the yoga of Action unfolds one's hidden potentials while preparing his psychological being to face and confront life's day to day activities.

Yogapathy

Now we presume that yogic principles and techniques when used in proper way can cure all types of ailments. That yogic system may be called **"Yogopathy".**

Considering it to be a system of therapy now we shall go into its various constituents and branches. These are:

1. Yogic Anatomy
2. Yogic Physiology
3. Yogic Pathology
4. Yogic Medicine

It is essential to have sound and complete knowledge of all these branches for treating a patient. All branches mentioned above are very vast and complicated. It is not possible to discuss them in great detail. However basic informations regarding all these will be given in this paper.

Yogic Anatomy

Our present knowledge of human body is based up on Gray's anatomy as taught in medical colleges and is only related to physical body. A human being is not a composite of skin, muscles, blood and bones but he possess three bodies. These are:

1. Physical-Sthool sharira
2. Astral-Shookshma sharira and
3. Causal-Karana sharira

For achieving goal of perfect health it is essential to render these three bodies devoid of ailments. A brief introduction of all these bodies would help us in understanding the problem of health and diseases.

Three bodies are grouped in five sheaths–Pancha kosha:

1. Annamaya kosha–Food sheath
2. Pranamaya kosha–Vital sheath
3. Manomaya kosha–Mental sheath
4. Vijnanmaya kosha–Intellect sheath and
5. Anandamaya kosha–Bliss sheath

Causal body is the inner most plane of a person. It is the source of astral and physical body. It is exclusively experienced in deep sleep and samadhi (higher form of super-consciousness). During the experience of joy or grief it is the causal body that operates. Its constituents are–**Avidya** (ignorance), **Asmita** (ego) and **Jivatma** (soul). Causal body and Anandamaya kosha are the same.

Astral body consists of three sheaths *e.g.*–vital, mental and intellectual. consiquently its ingredients are **intellect, mind, sense** and the **vital forces**. These vital force are known as **Pranas** that flows in astral tubes or **Nadis**. Prana is the subtlest form of energy that underlies all physical energies *e.g.* electricity, magnetism, light, heat etc. It also sustains all mental processes such as thinking, feeling, willing and reasoning. It is the sustainer of life and forces on this world.

In a restricted sense, prana is the vital force that sustains life of man by performing various vital functions and keeps the body alive. Breathing is as effect of the prana. It is linked to the mind and senses. Though prana is one, it is known by different names due to its different functions in the body. Accordingly there are five major pranas and five subpranas:

Pran, Apana, Samana, Vyana, and **Udana**–these are five main pranas. Naga, Kurma, Krikara, Devdatta and Dhanajaya–are five sub prans. Nadis are astral tubes through which pranic currents move. They can not be seen by naked eyes.

There are 72000 nadis. Among them **Ida, Pingala** and **Sushumna** are the most important. Entire astral body is permeated by a net work of these nadis. Ida and pingal correspond to left and right sympathetic chains. Ida flows through left nostril and is cooling. Pingala flows through the right nostril and is heating. Tamas predominates in ida, and Rajas in pingala.

Sushumna is the best of all nadis. It arises from the basal plexus and passes through the spinal column, through the subtle channel of the spinal cord, up to the crown of the head. Chakras are junctions where nadis cross over. All important chakras that are also very important mystic centres are situated in the sushumna. These are: **Muladhara, Swadhisthan, Manipur, Anahata, Vishudhi, Ajna** and **Shahastrar chakra**.

These three bodies are bound together by three knots–**granthis** and five afflictions–**Kleshas**. Three granthis are: **Karma granthi**–knot of Action, **Kama granthi**–knot of desire and **Avidya granthi**–Knot of ignorance. Centre of karma granthi is in physical body while astral and causal body are the centres for kama and avidya granthi. Five afflictions are: **Avidya**–ignorance, **Asmita**–ego principle, **Raga**–attachment, **Dwesh**–hatered and **Avinivesh**–clinginning to life or dread of death. Again these binding factors can be Tamasik, Rajasic or Satwik depending upon three gunas. Different constiuests of astral body are made up of **Tanmatras**–astral counter part of five elements *e.g.* Prithvi, Jal, Vayu and

Akash. Causal body projects astral body and then astral body becomes the basis for the physical body.

Physical body consists of food sheath that gives rise to flesh, bones, blood and nerves.

Yogic Physiology

All the physiological activities of three bodies can be grouped in following four categories:

1. Action: Which is of two types *a.* **Voluntary** and *b.* **Involuntary**. Again these can be of three types *i.* **Physical** *ii.* **Vocal** and *iii.* **Mental.**
2. Emotion
3. Will and
4. Wisdom

All types of actions mentioned above are not independent entity, rather there is intermingling to some extend *e.g.* there is some degree of action, will and wisdom in emotion and *vice versa.* Actions are seen to be performed by Jnanendriyas and karmendriyas but these are only instruments. There is no power in these organs to act independently.

On physical level all activities are supposed to be controlled by endocrinal and nervous system. Autonomic nervenous system regulates and governs most of our vital systems. Modern medical science has not been able to unreveal the mysteries of complex body mechanism. Up to certain stage physiologists know the process of metabolic activities. But how all these reactions test started are unknown to a great extent. And it will remain so as long as they are not able to peep beyond the physical body.

In reality all types of activities having originated from Supreme Self enter in different stratas of causal and astral bodies to reach the ultimate destination of physical plane as it were rays immersing from the sun travelling through different layers of space come to earth. Light is affected due to intermediate medium in sky. It is some thing like a light passing through a prism. If prism is colourless light passing through it would be unadulterated and come out in its original form. On the other hand if prism is coloured then original light would take up that colour and any one looking through it would see it in that colour. It is distorted and erroneous light. Similarly activities originating from Supreme Self get distorted due to intermediate medium of three bodies. Other activities such as emotion, will and wisdom also originate from the Supreme Self but get polluted due to intervening medium.

Entire biological functions are controlled and sustained by pranas. Without prana there would be no life on earth, there would be no existence of any object. Pranas keep body alive. Just as the queen bee is followed by the other bees and wherever the queen bee goes, there go all the bees, even so the senses and mind follow the movements of the pranas. If prana departs, the senses and mind also leave the body.

By control of prana, yogis have conquered death, they have mastered elements. They have performed various miracles. Control of prana enables a yogi to possess a dynamic personality. A brief account of various pranas, their centre and functions are given here:

Name	*Seat*	*Area of movement*	*Function*
1. Mukhya Prana	Heart	From heart to nostril	Respiration, converting food into vital food
2. Apana	Anus	From naval to feet	Excretion, exhalation
3. Samana	Naval	Entire body	Assimilation, distribution
4. Vyana	Above the root of generative organ	Entire body	Blood circulation
5. Udana	Throat	Up to head	Gives lightness to the body, separates astral form the physical body at the time of death.

Prana and apana are the main vital currents. The control of these two renders the functions of all other pranas harmonious.

Yogic Pathology

Similar to three bodies there are three basic pathologies too. Predominantly they operate in their corresponding bodies, but can manifest in any of the three. All pathogenic factors are actually modifications of only one pathology and that is ignorance–**Avidya**. However it is manifested at different planes assuming entirely different role. These are known as:

1. ***Mala:*** gross impurities on physical plane
2. ***Vikshepa:*** Distraction on astral plane and
3. ***Avarna:*** Veil on causal plane.

Mala can be detected or seen on physical level. It may manifest in the form of deformity or any type of defect in physical body. It is gross impurity. It may also manifest as gross defects in behaviour and personality. All those factors that are responsible for creating distraction of mind are grouped in vikshepa category. Avarna means a veil. It is the root of rest of two. Once it is eradicated other two are up rooted automatically.

These are responsible for creating intermediary factors that disort pure form of physiological activities. They give erroneous colour to all actions. They can be further classified in various subgroups depending up on gunas. Due to these pathological factors various types of distortions take place in all three bodies. However net effect of all of these pathogens is obstruction in free flow of pranic energy in nadis.

Once vital forces become disbalanced there is erratic functioning of autonomic and endocrinal system that lead to disturbance in chemical equilibrium and malfunctioning of different systems leading to manifestation of various diseases.

Afflictions affects functions of causal, astral and physical bodies. Avarna or veil is the pathological factor of the causal body, due to which one develops a feeling of separateness from the universal life and identifies oneself with the personality. Through ignorance one considers the perishable body to be the Atman or the Self.

This ignorance of one's essential nature leads to formation of various diseases of the mind. Fear is a cancer of the mind that corrodes the very vitals of it. Grief is tuberculosis. Greed is chronic anemia, pride is rheumatism. And thus all negative qualities of the mind are different forms of diseases making astral body distracted (vikshepa). Due to infestation of subtle body by greed, egoism, hatred, vanity, jealousy, wrath, selfishness, instable cravings for sense-enjoyments, one develops various granthis-knots and repeated experience of birth and death.

Diseases of the mind is called **Adhi**. Disease of the body is called **Vyadhi**. More than ninety percent of diseases are directly related to the psychic upset of the mind. The diseases of mind create agitation in the harmonious functioning of the pranas. Some nerves overwork, others do not work at all. Some cells and tissues overdo their work, others sit quite still and remain dull. This leads to development of toxins in the body.

Development of toxins in the body may or may not manifest in active diseases at once. They are potential diseases, and they must be removed.

It is important to understand how the energy of the spirit becomes limited by the impressions–**Samskaras** that are lodged in the unconscious. Just as a subterranean spring becomes polluted by the rocks through which it must pass, in the same way the energy of the soul becomes limited and polluted by the mental impressions of the unconscious.

Further again, the unfulfilled thoughts and desires continue to restrict the flow of vitality-prana proceeding from the mind. This results in disbalance in the humors of the body, and in course of time physical body becomes subject to various diseases and morbidities.

Today modern scientists and doctors are rediscovering the connections between mind and body and what is now called **"Psychosomatic medicine"** provides striking confirmation of the view held by ancient Rishis of India. It has been scientifically proved that well defined group of modern ailments like peptic ulcer, colitis, hypertension, allergic skin diseases, various types of arthritis, migraine and mental disorders are frequently initiated by emotional stresses. Sequence of events in development of various ailments can be summarised as follows:

Presence of ignorance (Avarna) leads to development of Panchakleshas which leads to malfunctions of mind. Mind has five important functions *e.g.* Right knowledge–**Pramana**, wrong knowledge–**Viparyay**, imagination–**Vikalpa**, memory–**Smriti** and sleep–**Nidra**. Disturbance in normal functions of mind cause various mental diseases (Vikshepa) that restrict the flow of Prana (vital forces) in the nadis (Astral channels). These astral channels–nadis are linked to the physical nervous system, and are controller of the chemical balance in the body. When prana do not flow in harmony in the body there is disbalance in **Kapha, Pitta**, and **Vayu**, there by all physiological activities such as respiration, circulation, metabolism and excretion are affected. When digestion and assimilation get affected body does not get proper nourishment. Due to defective function of excretory system toxins accumulate in blood stream. (Mala) A severe disbalance sets in all systems disturbing its equilibrium leading to exposure to various diseases.

It is important to note that although the three types pathological factors mentioned above may be primarily located in any one the three bodies but they are inter linked. One becomes the causative factor for intensification of other *e.g.* Mala primarily located in physical body may become originating factor for vikshepa or avarna or the *vice versa*. In this way any one of the three may trigger a process of developing rest of the two factors. In this way diseases of physical body can start or intensify diseases of astral or causal body and diseases of causal body may manifest predominantly is astral or physical body.

Yogic Medicine

All diseases are the modifications of only one disease *e.g.* **Avidya**–ignorance. Therefore aim of yogic medicine is to eradicate the root disease. On the basis of three types of pathologies predominantly active on three planes, diseases may be classified as:

1. Diseases rooted in the physical body
2. Diseases rooted in the astral body and
3. Diseases rooted in the causal body

Diseases that rooted in physical body will primarily require physical method of treatment. It includes all modes of treatments provided by modern medical science. Most of the diseases are beyond control or incurable by medicines because their root is in astral or causal body. For their eradication only astral and causal treatment would be effective.

It was stated before that although a disease may be primarily rooted in any of three bodies but its branches penetrate in other two, ultimately connected with root pathology that is Avarna. So adopting one mode of treatment will not serve the purpose. An integrated approach is needed. Physical mode of treatment is required to treat those diseases that are rooted in the physical body. While astral and causal approach is required to treat diseases that are basically rooted in those bodies. Yoga does not reject modern means of treatment. Human personality is a complex product of spirit and matter. There is no water tight distinction between the two. Actually matter is also the spirit in final analysis.

Therefore a careful and judicious approach is needed while treating a patient. Yoga therapist should not be hesitant in recommending physical mode of treatment while modern medical science should not ignore efficacy of astral and causal treatment e.g. yogic medicine. In other words modern modes of treatment is a part of Yogic medicine. We hope that one day all doctors will also be a yogi to treat a patient effectively.

Mode of Action of Yogic Medicine

Curative force is within every one. One is not cured by medicines, but by the life force itself, although medicine may assist in the removal of impediments. But too much dependence on medicine and medical drugs make one life devoid of strength and vitality. There is a source of infinite energy and vitality in every person.

Yogic medicine removes all impediments in the flow of pranas. Five afflictions–panchkleshas and three knots–granthis are main obstructions in natural flow of pranas. In restricted terms Mal, Vikshepa and Avarna are the real impediments. Yogic medicine is directed towards eradication of these three.

With decrease in the intensity of these, three bodies start getting proper vital energy, there by restoring their original purity. Health, happiness and experience of bliss depend upon this state of purity. The moment all these obstructions are removed one becomes free of mool vyadhi. Intermediary polluting factors are removed. Thus all physiological activities set in proper form giving perfect health, happiness, peace and person experiences Brahmananda the absolute bliss.

The Actual Treatment

It is very important to prepare body, mind and senses for receiving maximum benefit from yogic medicines. Faith and devotion–**Shradha** and **Vishwas** are two basic prerequisites. In other patients are benefited according to their faith and devotion. For this they must practice **Vahiranga sadhana** *e.g.* **Yama, Niyama, Asana, Pranayama** and **Pratyahar** till his **Antahkaran** and **Vahyakaran** is purified. **Ahimsa, Satyam, Brahmacharya, Asteya** and **Aparigrah** these are the five **Yamas** or restraints. **Shaucha, Santosh, Tapa, Swadhyaya** and **Ishwar pranidhana** these are the five **Niyamas** or observances.

Practice of asanas aid in personality integration and free flow of pranas. Breathing is an effect of the functions of the pranic energy. By regulating the breath, there is integration of the vital-physical aspect of personality. Pranayama consists of various exercises. Mind and prana are interdependent. The control of one leads to the control of the other. Mind sets up vibrations in the prana through its various desires and subtle inclinations. Then the pranic vibrations travel through numerous pranic channels in the astral body. The flow of pranic energy through the nadis is responsible for health and vitality of the physical body.

Pratyahar–withdrawal of the senses partly depends upon the control of prana and partly on the culture of mind. As the personality integrates the senses become obedient to the mind. Without this preparation there would be no any effect of yogic medicine. That is why many patients do not get any relief even after going through the course of yogic treatment.

After personality of a patient develops adequate sensitivity medicines for removing three pathological factors may be started.

Mala is eradicated by practice of **Nishkamya karma yoga**–seva, subha vichar and satsanga. Actions are unavoidable as long as one breathes. Prana or the vital forces, the mind and actions are related. By adopting a proper attitude towards oneself and the world, all actions become karma yoga. Any action thus performed is free from likes and dislikes, gain and loss and from the expectations of the fruit of action. In the perfected state of karma yoga, actions become the spontaneous overflow of the consciousness within us. **Affirmation, surrender,** and the feeling of **disassociation**–any one of these three may be developed to remove the bondage of karma **(Narayana bhava, Narayan arpan bhava and Nimitt bhava)**.

When a person affirms while doing action that he is one with karma then action becomes a wave in the consciousness. Action performed with the spirit of self-surrender to God or worship to God does not bind a person. It paves the way for the release of the soul because the result of such an action is not indentified with the subject.

Vikshepa can be destroyed by practice of **meditation**–dhyan and **upasana** *e.g.* practice of **Raj yoga** and **Bhakti yoga**. Individual mind is like a wave in the ocean of cosmic mind. When the vrittis of the mind are controlled and withdrawn the chitta reveals the natural of the Absolute Self-Atman. When a lake is calm, it reflects the vast sky. Yogic medicine aims to stop these thought waves. Practise of various limbs of yoga attenuate afflictions and finally burns them up through intuitive samadhi because these are the basis for the three types of karmas–good, evil, and mixed. Karmas are responsible for embodiment where one experiences all types of sufferings. When afflictions are destroyed karmas do not bear their fruits.

Negative thought-waves-**Klishta vrittis** can be destroyed by **Aklishta vrittis**–positive thought-waves. Anger by love, pride by humility, greed by generosity, craving by dispassion, and ignorance by knowledge. This method is known as **Pratipaksha bhawana**. Practice of **maitri, mudita, karuna** and **upeksha** are excellent qualities which increase the efficacy of yogic medicine.

Vikshepa can also be very effectively removed by adopting various techniques of **Samyam**–*e.g.* Dharna, Dyana and Samadhi. The focusing of the mind on one object, or on one thought form, is called concentration or **Dharna**. The continuity of this focused state deepens vision and insight–this is known as **Dhyana** wherein one perception continue to flow in a stream. When meditation is perfected one rises above the limited consciousness which supports the awareness of meditator, meditation and the object meditated up on and is led to the transcendental horizons of inner life. This is **Samadhi** which bestows profound insight, and leads to the intuitional realisation of the Self.

Along with practice of Raja yoga it is necessary to adopt various modes of upasana–Bhakti yoga. Devotion is of the nature of supreme love which expresses itself in ever increasing attachment to God. Just as a piece of iron is drawn to a magnet without any effort, in the same way, the spirit of a person is drawn to health, happiness and enlightenment when the obstructions are removed. There are five types of sentiments, which is satwic emotions when directed to properly, become effective tool for destroying vikshepa and providing liberation. They are:

1. **Shanta Bhawa:** The quiescent feeling of the heart for God–silent and secret.
2. **Dasya Bhawa:** A submissive attitude of love that exists between a servant and his master.
3. **Sakhya Bhawa:** A friendly familiarity of feeling, a heart to heart relation with God.
4. **Vatsalya Bhawa:** A tender, selfless devotion, as a mother's love for her child.

5. **Madhurya Bhawa**: Love for the sake of love; Supreme divinity becomes the beloved for the soul. There are many degrees and stages of above mentioned sentiments depending upon their intensity. These sentiments can be developed or intensified by practicing nine modes of devotion–**Navadha Bhakti**.

    1. **Shravana:** Listening to the stories of God.
    2. **Kirtan:** Singing divine glories. Expressing divine Love through thought, word and action.
    3. **Smarna:** Constant remembrance of God. Practice of meditation of God.
    4. **Padsevana:** Serving the Divine feet. The service of humanity is the service of Divine feet. Increasing awareness of the fact that it is God who underlies all beings, therefore, it is He who is being served through every action.
    5. **Archama:** Offering of flowers. It implies offering of flowers of virtue in the shrine of the heart.
    6. **Vandana**: Adoration of God in all. It is the increasing perception of the Divine Self in the world; and a consequent effacement of egoistic consciousness.
    7. **Dasya:** Submitting oneself to God.
    8. **Sakhyam:** A process of befriending God.
    9. **Atmanivedana:** Supreme surrender in God.

Adopting above methods of upasana one can eradicate vikshepa and mala effectively.

Avarna can be uprooted by adopting various techniques of **Jnana yoga** in which the individual soul works out its evolution, and final release, by exercising two-fold instruments–**Vahyakarana**–External instruments in the form of indriyas and **Antahkarna**–Internal instruments in the form of mind, intellect, ego, and subconscious. It is important to develop following qualities for getting benefit from Jnana yoga:

1. **Viveka:** Discriminative reason which shows the difference between the not-self (body, senses, mind and intellect) and the Self.

2. **Vairagya:** Dispassion. With the perception of illusoriness of the objects of the world, and mind develops increasing detachment towards them.
3. **Shatsampat:** Six fold treasure: *i.* **Shama** or serenity, *ii.* **Dama** or control of senses, *iii.* **Uparati** or renunciation of selfish actions, *iv.* **Titiksha** or endurance, *v.* **Shradha** or faith, *vi.* **Samadhana** or tranquility of mind.
4. **Mumukshuttwa:** Burning aspiration for Self-realization.

Actual practice of Jnana yoga medicine consists of the following stages:

1. **Shavana:** Listening to the teachings of vedantic philosophy for ascertaining the nature of the innermost Self as Brahman.
2. **Manan:** Reflection. It is reflective concentration of the nature of Self.
3. **Nididhyasana:** Meditation on the Self wherein the mind assumes its intuitive functions of Brahmakar vritti and begins to reflect the absolute, with increasing expansion and luminosity.
4. **Nirvikalpa samadhi** and **Sakshatkara:** Intense meditation leads to the development of nirvikalpa samadhi wherein the Self is realised as distinguished from the three bodies and five sheaths, the basis of this world-process. Nirvikalpa samadhi bestows Sakshatkara or Self-realisation by removing the veil of ignorance-Avarna.

In short, essence of Yogic medicine is the practice of integral yoga–a synthesis of Karma yoga, Bhakti yoga, Raj yoga and Jnana yoga along with preparatory practice of Yama, Niyam, Asana, Pranayam and Pratyahara. When one is free of Mala, Vikshepa and Avarna all three knots of heart–Avidya granthi, Karma granthi and Karma granthi are destroyed and he attains liberation from all limitations including all ailments affecting three bodies.

Scientific Studies Giving Insight in Efficacy of Yogopathy

According to several recent reports published in news media and professional journals it has been established beyond doubt that spirituality can be influential in contributing to total well being.

A conference on spirituality and healing sponsored by Harvard Medical School in December 1995 attended by 1000 physicians and scholars. President of Harvard's Mind/Book Medical Institute presented results of several years of research.

According to Dr. Benson, one of the most effective methods for eliciting relaxation and facilitating physical healing is regular meditational practice. He has found the meditation is helpful in overcoming insomnia, improving female fertility, and reducing hypertension to normal levels in most people. He concluded that underlying cause of up to nine-tenths of the symptoms and diseases that bring people to physicians is stress that increases blood pressure, pulse, and breathing rate. He and many other physicians, now teach their patients meditation and japa for twenty minutes a day.

Several year ago, a study of 91000 people in the rural area of the state of Maryland indicated that individuals who had a religious orientation or regularly attended church services of their choice, were healthier. In contrast to those with no religious or spiritual base. They lived longer and had a much lower incidence of heart disease, cirrhosis of the liver, and lung problems.

A 1989 article in the journal of religion and Health describing a survey funded in part the University of North Carolina and the Duke University Medical Center revealed that men ages 55 and over with spiritual values have diastolic blood pressure 6 mm lower than those who said faith is only some what or not important to them.

A study published in a 1988 edition of the Southern Medical Journal reported that, in a San Francisco Hospital, 201 coronary patients who had no one praying for them were twice as likely to suffer congestive heart failure than those prayed for by people who did not even know them, and were four times as likely to have a heart attack.

A Word of Caution

It is not necessary that all patients will get equal benefit. There is a limiting factor having major role to play in this regard. That is the law of karma. Every Yoga therapist and patient must be well aware of this divine law. Important aspects of law of karma that are related to yogic medicine are very briefly discussed here.

All types of experiences are the resultant of one's own action. All actions performed by mind, speech and body produce subtle impressions known as **Sanskaras** are accumulated in unconscious mind. Some of these impressions may fructify immediately, or some time later in this embodiment or it may take several births for its fructification. There are three types of karmas:

1. **Kriyaman karma**–Present action
2. **Prarabdha karma**–Fructifying action and
3. **Sanchit karma**–Accumulated action

Actions being done in the present moment are called kriyaman karma. Karmas that are fructifying in this life are Prarabdh karma, and karma that is coming from previous lives or that would fructify in future embodiments are called accumulated karmas.

Prarabdha karma is in restricted sense determine **Ayu**-age, **Bhoga**-experience of pleasure or pain and **Jati**-class. These can't be changed by any of present effort. However effort that is being done for the change appear to have gone wasted without producing any positive result. But it is not so according to law of karma. All actions must produce its result accordingly even if results are not seen immediately.

Thus it is possible that some patients may not get desired result from any treatment due to their prarabdha karma. Therefore it is prime responsibility of yoga therapist to prepare such patients spiritually and mentally to bear sufferings with the sense of surrender and austerity. It is advisable to continue treatment with yogic medicine so that their shubha sanskaras- auspicious impressions intensify.

It is very important to explain to all patients that a person is not limited to his life only. But he is a eternal traveller to immortality. No one comes on this earth as a blank sheet but every one brings a big bundle of his previous karmas and writes some new stories in present life making it more heavier. This goes on till he is enlightened.

A person when becomes enlightened though acting, does not act, though thinking he is not caught in the waves of thoughts, though desiring, he is beyond desires, though wishing to live, he is beyond mortality, though trying to perfect himself, he is the very essence of perfection, though seemingly delighting in the objects of the world he is the very embodiment of bliss. Though expressing concern towards day to day developments, he is beyond grief; and is established in the experience of unending satisfaction. This is the state of Jeevan mukta–the goal of every individual.

Yoga as a System of Psychotherapy

P.V. Krishna Rao

The concepts and methods of yoga have become an integral part of Indian philosophico-religious thought soon after their formulation and systematization (Eliade, 1969; Werner, 1977). They have also found a prominent place in the ancient medicinal system of *Ayurveda* which advocated yoga for cure and prevention of physical and mental diseases (Dasgupta, 1975, Kuppuswamy, 1985). Thus, over centuries in philosophical, religious and medical contexts yoga has been a living tradition in India.

The curiosity of scientists in the claims of yogis, the counter cultural movements in the United States of America and a general shift in the Western zeitgeist precipitated by wars, scientific developments, rampant social and psychological problems led to a serious examination of Eastern thought and practices by the West in the early 20th century.

This soon contributed to a proliferation of research studies, articles and books on Indian concepts, traditions and technique. The religious personalities such as Maharshi Mahesh Yogi and Swami Rama, among others helped scientists to undertake a fair and systematic investigation of the claims associated with yogic practices in the later half of the present century. As a result of this, yoga gained prominence as a psychophysiological system of self-regulation with therapeutic implications. The humanistic and transpersonal approaches in contemporary psychology facilitated the recognition of the relevance of yoga for health, well being and enhancement of human potential. Meditative practices have come to be identified as adjuncts to psychotherapy (*e.g.*, Deatherage 1975; Engler, 1984) and as metatherapies (*e.g.*, Goleman, 1971). In India religious traditions, organizations and personalities–the gurus and god-men have always been fulfilling the psychotherapeutic needs of countless people through one or the other yogic methods. Psychologists and psychiatrists who were discontented with the application of western psychotherapeutic concepts and tools in the Indian context have been looking into their heritage for appropriate leads (Akhilananda, 1952, Singh, 1977, Satyanand, 1972, Vijaya-lakshmi, Vindhya Sudhakar, Kalpana Rao, 1986). Nevertheless, the attempts to formulate and develop a psychotherapeutic system out of yoga in a way characteristic of science have been strikingly meager. Theories and concepts that are based on observation and hypothesis, and techniques that are verified and found useful in clinical practice only would lead to the development of a school of psychotherapy. The system of yoga presents certain formidable problems for such endeavors.

Yoga is found embedded in various context–from philosophico-religious and divine to magico-occult and diabolical. Accordingly it refers to certain world views-metaphysical conceptions concerning man and universe, certain life styles, attitudes and values and psycho-physiological practices. In adapting yogic concepts and methods for psychotherapeutic purposes, one has to decide to what extent one subscribes to the metaphysics of the system. Removing or isolating the tools and concepts of yoga from their context and using them in therapy requires justification. That they are age old and traditional cannot suffice. Any justification ought to come from scientific theorization based on experimentation and clinical practice.

A significant attempt in the direction of formulating and developing yoga as a psychotherapeutic system was made in recent years by Swamy Rama and his disciples at the Himalayan International Institute of Yoga Science and Philosophy in the United States. Though not completely free from metaphysical commitments and personal predilections, *Yoga and psycho-theraphy : The evolution of consciousness* of Swamy Rama,

Ballantine and Swamy Ajaya (1976) and *Psychotherapy east and west : A unifying paradigm* of Swamy Ajaya (1984) present a strong case for yoga as a system of psychotherapy and describes it in some detail. Their system is based on *samkhya-yoga, hatha yoga, advaita vedanta* and *tantra*. From their account it appears that those of us who are looking for a conceptual framework and a set of procedures close to the Indian mind would certainly find an alternative in Yoga.

Psychologists and other professional in the areas of mental health and hygiene may adapt yoga as a psychotherapeutic system as a general conceptual framework like other schools of psychotherapy such as psychoanalysis or rational emotive therapy. Or they may use yoga theory and techniques when appropriate as a part of an eclectic approach. Such an adaptation must be based on contemporary interpretation of classical ideas from a psychological perspective and current research on yoga practices. Further, yoga psychotherapy should not involve itself with any religion, deity, spiritual leader or order. Spiritual issues need be their concern only when the client brings them to be session. The content of each session should originate from the client, his needs and issues.

At the present stage of evolution of yoga as a psychotherapeutic system it is desirable to use yoga in the general framework of psychotherapy. The experiential basis of psychotherapy, namely, the psychological contact between the therapist and the client must be the same as that of conventional humanistic therapies. The vehicle of interaction must be the face to face interview between the two. Yoga may be introduced as a procedure of self-mastery involving behavioural techniques and introspection. Nevertheless, yoga psychotherapy which combines yogic concepts and techniques and psychotherapy need not stop with self-mastery, it also should aim at mastering the environment unlike traditional yoga.

As a holistic system it deals with the body, mind and behaviour in a synergistic way. For this purpose it makes use of the procedures of asanas, mudras, breathing, relaxation, visualization and meditation and the principles of yoga such as *yama (satya, ahimsa, asteya, brahmacharya, aparigraha), niyama (soucha, santosha, tapas, svadhyaya, Iswarapranidhana), maitri, karuna, mudita, upeksha, abhyasa, vairagya, nishkama karma,* to mention a few. Learning and working with some of these principles may be a part of the process.

The general orientation of yoga therapy must be that the client should develop a broader perspective on self and world, self discipline, responsibility, acceptance, congruence, compassion and an attitude of witness to life with less ego involvement and more task orientation. From a psychological perspective meditation is essentially a procedure of expanding one's awareness and directing that awareness to achieve control over body, mind, feelings and emotions, thoughts and behaviour. An attitude of meditation in action, characterized by attention, awareness and volitional control enables the individual to think, emote and act for self-fulfillment and social harmony must be the goal of yoga psychotherapy (Ajaya, 1984).

The yoga therapist must be a role model to the client and cultivate in himself all the characteristics that are considered necessary for helping professionals in humanistic or other circles (Egan, 1982). However, the yoga psychotherapist need not pretend that he is a guru or a fully enlightened person but merely another person seeking freedom from suffering and to realize his potentialities for growth.

As yoga embraces all aspects of human life and also provides techniques for the regulation of the mind-body complex, it is up to the researchers and clinicians to develop an indigenous psychotherapeutic system out of it, which would be comprehensive enough to deal with the complexities of modern life and its cultural milieu.

References

1. Ajaya, Swamy (1984), *Psychotherapy east and west: A unifying paradigm,* Honsedale: Himalayan International Institute of Yoga Science and Philosophy.
2. Akhilananda, S. (1952), *Mental Health and Hindu Psychology,* London: George Allen and Unwin.

3. Dasgupta, S. (1975), *A History of Indian Philosophy*, Vol. 2, Delhi: Motilal Banarsidas.
4. Deatherage, G. (1975), Clinical use of mindfulness meditation technique in short term psychotherapy, *Journal of Transpersonal Psychology*, 7, 133-143.
5. Eagan, G. (1982), *The Skilled Helper*, Monterey: Brooks/cole Publishing Company.
6. Eliade, M. (1969), *Yoga: Immortality and freedom*, Princeton: Princeton University Press.
7. Engler, J. (1984), Therapeutic aims in psychotherapy and meditation: Developmental stages in the representation of self, *Journal of Transpersonal Psychology*, 16, 25-61.
8. Goleman, D. (1971), Meditation as meta therapy: Hypothesis towards a proposed 5th state of consciousness, *Journal of Transpersonal Psychology*, 31, 1-26.
9. Kuppuswamy, B. (1985), *Elements of Ancient Indian Psychology*, New Delhi: Vani Educational Books.
10. Rama, Swamy, Ballentine, R., and Ajaya, Swamy (1976), *Yoga and Psychotherapy: The Evolution of Consciousness*. Honesdale: Himalayan Institute of Yoga Science and Philosophy.
11. Satyanand, D. (1972), *Dynamic Psychology of the Gita of Hinduism*, New Delhi: Oxford and IBH.
12. Singh, H.G. (1977), *Psychotherapy in India*, Agra: National Psychological Corporation.
13. Vijayalakshmi, S., Vindhya Sudhakar, U., and Kalpana Rao, V. (1986), Role of a counsellor in the Indian context, *Journal of Indian Psychology*, 5, 76-82.
14. Werner, K. (1977), *Yoga and Indian Philosophy*, Delhi: Motilal Banarsidass.

Yoga for Stress Management

A.M. Moorthy

Meaning : Stress is the body's physical, mental and chemical reaction to circumstance that frighten, excite, confuse, challenge, surprise, anger, endanger or irritate. The events that cause stress may be good or bad.

Definition : Stress can be defined as a state that occurs when people are faced with demands from the environment that require them to change in some way.

Stress may be due to environmental, physical or psychological.

The stress producing circumstances or conditions are known as "stressors". There is no "Psychological stress" without physiological involvement.

The general response, or the General Adaptation Syndrome (GAS) consists of three stages:

a. The Alarm Reaction

b. The Resistance Stage

c. The Exhaustion Stage

One man's stress may be another man's pleasure.

Reactions to Stress

- More blood sugars and fats flow to the muscle and brain.
- Heart rate increases.

- Breathing becomes faster.
- Many muscles tense and tighten.
- Blood pressure rises.
- Stomach and intestines temporarily halt digestion.
- Perspiration increases.
- Blood clotting mechanisms start up.
- All senses are heightened.

Stress Load Symptoms–Too Little Stress

- Dull thinking
- Irritability
- Decreased motivation
- Lethargic performance
- Negativity
- Erratic interrupted sleep
- Poor quality performance.

The Right Amount of Stress

- Clear thinking and perception
- High motivation
- High energy and expectations
- Effective decision making and problem analysis
- Excellent memory
- High creativity
- Normal sleep patterns.

Too Much Stress

- Cloudy thinking
- Irritability
- Motivated but overloaded
- Poor quality performance
- Chronic fatigue

- Social withdrawal
- Decreased creativity.

An estimated 50 to 80% of all diseases in this country have stress related origins. A specific list of diseases that may be stress induced covers from head to toe.

Migraise Headaches : Headaches due to abnormal blood flow in the arteries of the blood.

Hypertension : High blood pressure.

Bronchial Asthma : Recurrent attacks of shortness of breath and wheezing due to spasming contractions of the lungs.

Peptic Uleer : A defect or hole in the living of the esophagus, stomach or first portion of the small intestine that is caused by excess digestive acid.

Coronory Artery Disease : Heart disease.

Amenorrhea : Absence or abnormal stoppage of the menstrual cycle.

Sleep Onset Insomnia : Difficulty falling to sleep.

Enuresis : Bed wetting.

Drug Addiction

Alcoholism

Stress occurs when a person is faced with environmental demands, whether pleasant or unpleasant, that require some kind of adjustments or adaptation. Traumatic events are extremely stressful situations involving grave physical risk. Life events are changes that disrupt people's usual activities.

How to Evaluate the Stress

Personal Stress Inventory

1. Did you now or ever have you had?

Yes	*No*	
–	–	High blood pressure (Hypertension)
–	–	Heart trouble
–	–	Colitis (irritated inflamed intestine)
–	–	Ulcer or digestion trouble
–	–	Asthma
–	–	Cancer
–	–	Arthritis

2. To what extent do you experience the following, using the following scale?

   1. Never, 2. Rarely, 3. Sometimes, 4. Often, 5. Always.

1	*2*	*3*	*4*	*5*	
–	–	–	–	–	Sweaty palms
–	–	–	–	–	Cold hands and feets
–	–	–	–	–	Tension headaches
–	–	–	–	–	Teeth grinding
–	–	–	–	–	Neck pains
–	–	–	–	–	Uncontrollable muscle spasms
–	–	–	–	–	Pain in the shoulder
–	–	–	–	–	Poor quality sleep
–	–	–	–	–	Chronic fatigue

How frequently do you experience the following:

1	*2*	*3*	*4*	*5*	
–	–	–	–	–	Trouble concentrating
–	–	–	–	–	Anxiety
–	–	–	–	–	Irritability
–	–	–	–	–	Job dissatisfaction
–	–	–	–	–	Depression
–	–	–	–	–	Decision making anxiety
–	–	–	–	–	Stressful dreams

– – – – – Pessimism

– – – – – A short-fused temper

Muscle Tension Evaluation

Severe stress frequently produces very tender points in some of the muscles. These bands of muscle tension are called trigger points or knots.

Breathing Evaluation

The way you breath is a good indicator of your state of stress. By evaluating five breathing factors you can tell if stress has interrupted your body's oxygen intake and waste gas elimination. They are:

a. Length of inhalation

b. Length of exhalation

c. Shoulder elevation

d. Action of the diaphragm

e. Overall control

Posture Evaluation

Check the picture that most closely resembles your posture. Often, poor posture indicates stress, while simultaneously contributing to it.

Forward Head

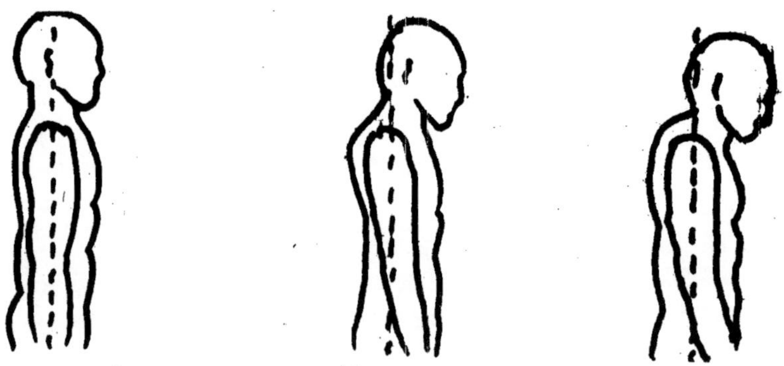

Normal Posture ***Mild*** ***Severe***

Round Shoulders

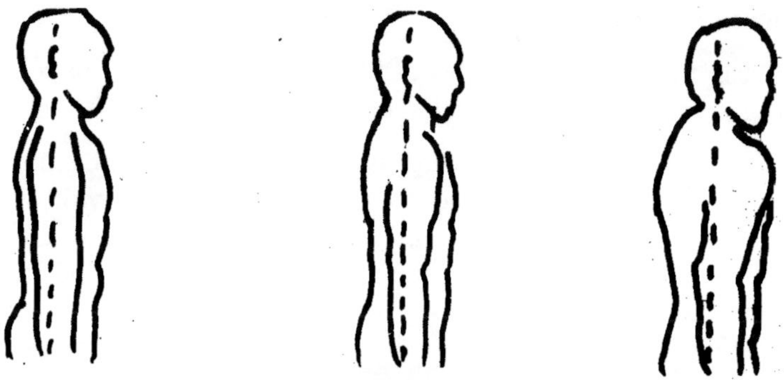

Normal Posture *Mild* *Severe*

Elevated Shoulder

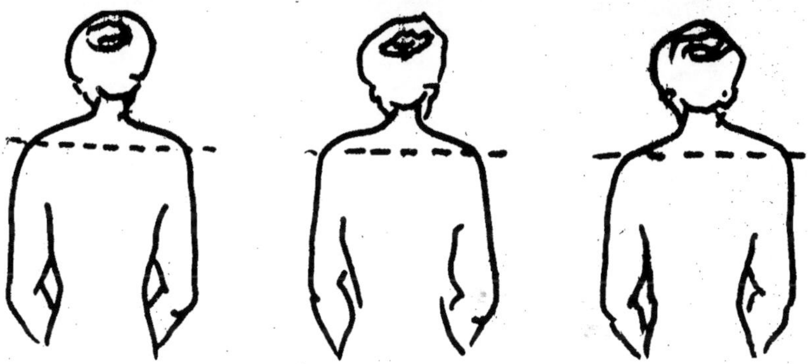

Normal Posture *Mild* *Severe*

Lordosis (Pelvic or Sway Back)

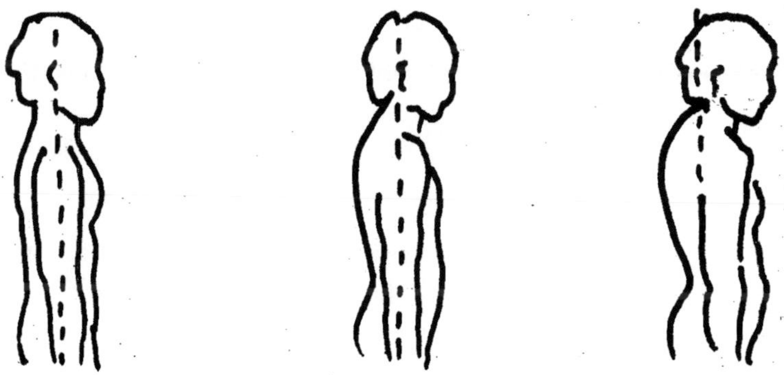

Normal Posture *Mild* *Severe*

Flexibility Evaluation

Excess tightness in muscles can cause poor posture, pain and fatigue, as well as joint and skeletal problems.

Ex. Round shoulders are usually caused by tight muscles on the front of the chest and shoulder out of balance with weak muscles on the back between the shoulder blades (the rhomboids and middle and lower trapezius).

Developing an Anti-Stress Plan
Stress Reduction Reference Chart

Problems	*Stress Reduction Technique*
1. High Blood Pressure	Controlled breathing, aerobic and flexibility exercises, deep relaxation and diet.
2. Colitis	Deep relaxation and breathing exercises.
3. Ulcer and digestive trouble	Controlled breathing, aerobic exercises and deep relaxation.
4. Asthma	Breathing mechanics, abdominal strengthening exercises, posture and stretching exercises.
5. Cancer	Controlled breathing, flexibility and aerobic exercises, deep relaxation.
6. Arthritis	Flexibility and posture improvement exercises.
7. Depression	Deep relaxation training
8. Heart trouble	Controlled breathing, flexibility exercises (mild) deep relaxation (yogic) and mild yogic diet.

Stress Measurement
Social Readjustment Rating Scale

Life Event	*Mean LEM value*
Death of spouse	100
Divorce	73
Merital separation	65
Jail term	63
Death of close family member	63
Personal injury or illness	53
Marriage	50
Pregnancy	40
Sex difficulties	35
Change in financial status	38
Death of close friend	37
Trouble with in-laws	29
Outstanding personal achievements	28
Change in living conditions	25
Merital reconciliation	45
Retirement	45
Change in living condition	25
Change in sleeping habits	16
Change to different line of work	36

Coping with Stress

Many coping patterns that are used to eliminate a general psychological response elicited by most stressors-anxiety. It is used to refer to symptoms of psychopathology to realistic features, to irrational emotional status, and to normal reactions experienced by everyone.

People with stress tend to be impatient, aggressive, competitive. The following are the symptoms of behaviour:

- moving, eating or walking rapidly.
- Hurrying the ends of sentences.
- Impatience.
- Feeling guilty about relaxation.
- Not listening to the opinion of others.
- Relating success to time *i.e.*, speed is everything.

The group or individual stress can be tackled by the techniques of behaviour modification or behaviour therapy. It is a discipline, a unique orientation to the therapeutic treatment of behavioural problems.

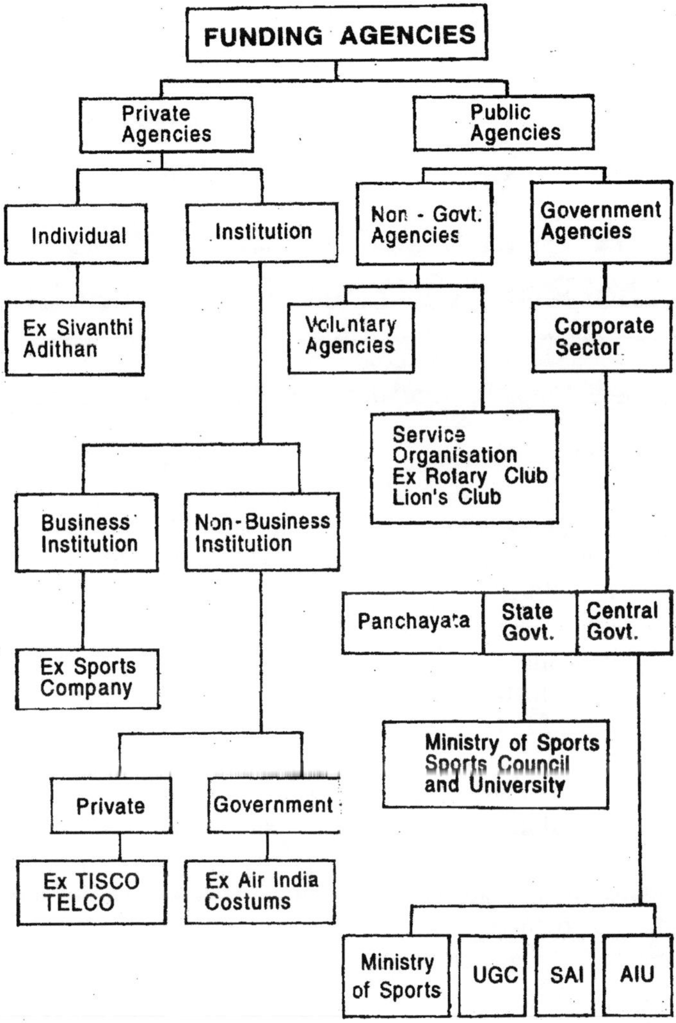
FUNDING AGENCIES
Private Agencies
Public Agencies
Individual
Institution
Non - Govt. Agencies
Government Agencies
Ex Sivanthi Adithan
Voluntary Agencies
Corporate Sector
Service Organisation Ex Rotary Club Lion's Club
Business Institution
Non-Business Institution
Panchayata
State Govt.
Central Govt.
Ex Sports Company
Ministry of Sports Sports Council and University
Private
Government
Ex TISCO TELCO
Ex Air India Costums
Ministry of Sports
UGC
SAI
AIU

Latent Autoimmune Diabetes Mellitus (LADA) : A Challenge for the Future : The Role of Yoga for Prevention

S.C. Jain, B. Talukdar, Girish Jha & Alkallppal

The World Health Organization Expert Committee (WHO) on Diabetes Mellitus (1) and The National Diabetes Data Group (NDDG), (2) recommended that the term 'Mature–onset' and adult-onset diabetes mellitus be replaced by non-insulin-dependent diabetes mellitus (on Type 2 diabetes) with subcategories of non-obese and obese. However, Type 2 diabetes is heterogenous and while a substantial number of patients are obese and hyper-insulinaemic/many diabetics often have insulin hyposecretion and treatment fails with oral hypoglycemic drugs. Accordingly, subjects in this non-obese group could actually have Type 1, diabetes, in a slowly evolving form. A number of epidemological studies of adult diabetes patients show that over 14% were insulin-treated. The clinical onset of diabetes is usually less acute in adult patients, so leading to an initial diagnosis of Type 2 diabetes and there is a group of patients, hitherto labelled as 'Type 1' 1/2 diabetes who are non-obese, and initially may be treated as Type 2 diabetes, yet progress rapidly to insulin dependency, within months or a few years of diagnosis.

Patients reported as 'Type 1 1/2 diabetes' show some of the classical features of Type 1 diabetes including weight loss, low C-peptide concentrations, an increased frequency of HLA DR3 and DR4, and positive tests for islet cell antibodies (ICA) (1) The RIA insulin assay may not be very helpful in the early diagnosis this sub-group. Recently, a high frequency of antibodies to glutamic acid decarboxylase (anti-GAD) has been reported in these patients and anti-GAD assay is now considered to be very useful for their identification. Therefore, 'Type 1 1/2 diabetes' is likely to be a slowly-evolving Type 1 diabetes and a name latent autoimmune diabetes of adults (LADA) has been suggested to describe such patients and assay for anti-GAD would be a valuable tool for prediction of insulin dependency. A review of studies conducted on the relationship between NIDDM, glucose intolerance, insuline action, obesity and weight gain, revealed that *(i)* majority of Type 2 diabetes are obese and or hyperinsulinaemic; *(ii)* Pre-existing insuline resistance is one of the important contributing factor for development of impaired glucose tolerance (IGT) and diabetes: *(iii)* aging and physical inactivity are other possible precipitating factors. We have previously identified the demographic and biochemical characteristics of Type 2 diabetics who respond to yoga therapy. These group of subjects after a short term yoga practice alone (without any modification in diet and caloric intake and without any hypoglycemic drugs), showed a significant decrease in blood glucose levels, improvement in glucose tolerance and a decrease in diabetic severity scale index (Table 1 and 2).

Another-study showed that yoga practice resulted in a significant decrease WHR (Waist-Hip ratio), AIT (Area index total under glucose tolerance curve) and glycated haemoglobin in middle aged non-insulin dependent diabetics (Table 3). This study provides an indirect evidence for the improved insulin responsiveness or decrease in insulin-resistance in this group of patients by yoga.

It is now well documented that patients with high blood pressure, as a group, are resistant to insulin-mediated glucose uptake and are hyperinsulinaemic when compared to a closely-matched population with normal blood pressure. These abnormalities persist despite successful drug treatment for hypertension. These studies indicate a close association of

Table 1

Blood Glucose Levels (Fasting, OGT man) and Area Index Total (AIT) of NIDDM Patients of Various Response Groups, Before (B) and After (A) Yoga therapy

Parameter Poor Response (n=45)	*Group I Fair Response (n=28)*	*Group II Good Response (n=76)*	*Group III (n=149)*	*All subjects*
Fatting blood				
Glucose (mg/dl)				
(B)	176.3±62.7	136.6±42.3	109.7±21.8	134.8±38.0
(A)	131.5±43.2*	96.6±19.8*	93.7±14.1*	100.9±23.9*
OGT_{max}(mg/dl)				
(B)	348.3±66.7	273.6±57.3	227±46.3	272.2±545
(A)	274±52.5**	196.7±9.2*	158.5±9.6**	200.44±22.5*
AIT				
Glucose mg. h'dl				
(B)	1159±246	931±181	767±150	915±184
(A)	880±213**	643±103*	508±77**	645±122
SSI				
(B)	2.66±0.80	1.89±0.67	1.39±0.59	1.86±0.6
(A)	1.72±0.70*	0.89±0.49*	0.46±0.55	0.98±0.6

Value are mean ± S.D. AIT=area index total in glucose tolerance test: OGT_{max}=blood glucose max in oral glucose tolerance test, SSI=severity scale index derived from normal values of AIT=B5A-**P<0.01*, ***P<0.001.*

diabetes-hypertension and insulin resistance and Talukdar and Jain reported that yoga practice provides a protection against oxidative stress (free radicals) damage to cell membrane integrity and increases the erythrocyte cell membrane Na^+ K^+ ATPase activity (Table 4). ATP sensitive K^+ channels in the cell membrane are now thought to be mediate glucose-induced beta cell insulin release. It is now evident that yoga can provide an alternative non-pharmacological mode of treatment and management of Type-2 patients. Our recent studies (WHO sponsored project) indicate that yoga modulates insulin responsiveness to glucose load in both Type 1 and Type 2 diabetics (unpublished).

Table 2

Characteristics of 30 Non-Insulin Dependent Diabetes Mellitus (NIDDM) patients before (B) and After (A) Yoga Training

	Mean±S.D	
Variables	*(B)*	*(A)*
Age (years)	59.5±6.71	
Duration of disease (years)	17.0±5.85	
BMI (Kg/m²)	22.5±2.14	21.9±2.40
WHR	0.870±0.056	0.853±0.059*
Caloric Intake (kcal/day)	1631±265	1657±237
Fasting Blood Glucose (mg/dl)	14.23±41.3	10.49±39.3*

BMI=Body Mass Index, WHR=Waist-hip ratio.

*$p < 0.01$, B Vs A.

Recent studies confirm that a substantial population of patients perhaps upto 20% with an onset of diabetes in a adult life have a slow onset of Type 1 diabetes with autoimmune features: this group is termed as latent autoimmune diabetes of adult (LADA). The natural history of LADA is predictable on clinical grounds and from results of ICA and C-peptide but availability of laboratory assay for anti-GAD provides for a specific discrimination of these patients for clinical management. However, the challenge for diabetologists, yoga researchers and yoga therapists seems to device therapy protocol which will allow preservation of insulin secretion and pancreatic beta cell function in LADA patients.

Table 3

Blood Glucose Area Index Total (AIT), Glycated Haemoglobin (GHb), Plasma Triglycerides (TG), Total Cholesterol (TC) and High Density Lipoproteins-cholesterol (HDL-C) values, Before (B) and After (A) Yoga Training

	Mean±S.D	
Variables	*(B)*	*(A)*
AIT (mgh/dl)	943±187	787±163*
GHb (%)	11.2±1.51	9.3±1.62**
TG (mg/dl)	116.4±27.9	106±19.7**
TC (mg/dl)	214.4±32.6	201.7±18.5*
HDL-C	48.7±9.1	54.3±10.4**
SSI	1.93±0.68	0.98±0.56

*p<0.01, **p<0.05, B Vs A

SSI=Severity scale index derived from AIT.

A review of study data on clinical features of insulin-treated diabetes mellitus (ITDM) and Type 2 diabetes in relation to anti-GAD status (Table 5 and 6) shown the distinctive features for identification and appropriate treatment.

Selection of Patients and Results

The study was conducted on 65 adult patients with diabetes in adulthood. All the patients were initially treated with diet alone or oral hypoglycemic drugs, but in whom the diagnosis of Type 1 versus Type 2 diabetes was not clear cut on clinical grounds. The selection criteria included > 30 years of age at diagnosis, absence of Ketouria, and with no apparent need for insulin treatment for atleast 6 months after initial diagnosis. Insulin therapy was initiated on clinical grounds in 19 patients, while 46 subjects remained on diet alone and or oral hypoglycemic agent(s) with acceptable metabolic control.

The ITDM differed from the Type 2 diabetes group according to number of features (Table 5), including a lower mean age (p<0.02), a lower age at onset of diabetes (p<0.002), a lower mean body weight, and a lower mean serum C-peptide concentration (p<0.001). Moreover, the mean level on anti-GAD

Table 4

Physical characteristics of hypertensive and normotensive subject before (B) and after (A) yoga training

	Hypertensive subject (n=30)		*Normote Ive subjects (n=30)*	
	(B)	*(A)*	*(B)*	*(A)*
Age (yrs)	48.5±11.7	-	47.1±11.2	-
Duration (yrs)	7.6±5.3	-		-
B.M.I. (kg/M²)	22.4±3.5	21.9±3.0	21.9±3.8	205±3.7
S.B.P. (mmHg)	149.7±14.0	135.5±11.3*	122.6±16.2	118.6±18.4
D.B.P. (mmHg)	99.2±9.0	86.9±5.1*	76.5±6.8	72.4±7.4
H.R. (Beats/min)	74.7±18.5	70.6±16.5	73.2±9.5	69.3±7.5
6 MD (Meters)	479.0±85.0	519.0±86.0*	542.0±45.0	560.0±32.0

Value are Mean ± SD, B.M.I.=Body Mass Index, S.B.P.=Average (one week) resting systolic blood pressure, D.B.P.=Average (one week) resting diastolic blood pressure, H.R.+Average (one week) Heart rate, 6 MD=Distance in meters walked in six minutes. *P<0.01, B Vs A.

Table 5

Changes in plasma lipids, erythrocyte lipid peroxidation and $Na^+ K^+$ ATPase activity in hypertensive and normotensive subjects before (B) and after (A) yoga

	Hypertensive subject (n=30)		*Normote Ive subjects (n=30)*	
	(B)	*(A)*	*(B)*	*(A)*
Plasma triglycerides (mg/dl)	121.0õ22.5	98.0õ16.4*	74.0õ19.3[a]	69.0õ16.4[a]
Plasma cholesterol (mg/dl)	228.0õ24.5	214.0õ17.5*	193.0õ34.4[b]	178.0õ21.4*[b]
Plasma HDL-cholesterol (mg/dl)	52.4õ9.3	58.3õ3.6*	67.8õ6.3[b]	66.1õ5.1[b]
Lipid peroxidation (nmol/ml of RBC)	1.98õ0.43	1.32õ0.31*	1.04õ0.27[a]	0.94õ0.26[b]
Na* K* ATPase activitay (umol pi/mg protein/hr)	0.18õ0.03	0.22õ0.03*	0.35õ0.03[a]	0.36õ0.32[b]

Value are Mean õ SD, *$p<0.01$, B Vs. A.

a=$p<0.01$; b=$p<0.05$ (Hypertensive Vs. Normotensive subjects).

was 66.8+10.2 units, significantly higher than for the Type 2 diabetes group 9.9+1.9 units ($p<0.001$) and respective frequencies of positive test for anti-GAD were 74% (14/19) versus 4.3% (2/46).

Table 6

Characteristics of Patients with Insulin Treated Diabetes Mellitus (ITDM) and Those with Type 2 Diabetes

	ITDM	*Type 2 Diabetes*	*P*
n	19	46	
Age (Yr)	47.2±2.2	53.5±1.4	0.02
Duration of Diabetes (Yr)	11.0±1.9	8.6±0.9	NS
Weight (Kg.)	61.3±3.5	68.6±2.3	NS
C-Peptide (ug ml^{-1})	1.3±0.38	4.6±0.37	<0.001
Ant-GAD (Units)	66.8±10.2	9.9±1.9	<0.001
Frequency of anti-GAD positivity	73.7%	4.3%	<0.001

Results are mean±SEM

Table 7

Characteristics of Patients with 'Adult Onset' Diabetes in Relation to Anti-GAD Status

Parameters	*Anti-GAD Units*		
	GAD^{+}	*GAD^{-}*	*P*
Number	16	49	
Age (Yr)	46.6±2.7	53.3±1.3	0.021
Duration of Diabetes (Yr)	7.8±1.5	9.7±1.0	NS
Weight (Kg.)	59.1±3.3	68.9±2.3	0.021
C-Peptide (ug ml^{-1})	1.3±0.4	4.3±0.4	<0.001
Anti-GAD (Units)	84.3±8.0	7.7±0.5	<0.001
Diet	0.0	8.2	<0.001
Oral Agents	12.5	81.6	<0.001
Insulin	87.5	10.2	<0.001

Results are Mean±SEM

Attributes of subjects who gave positive or negative tests for anti-GAD are shown in Table 6; distribution of these values for these indices in similar to that for ITDM and Type 2 diabetes groups, respectively. Recently Zimmet *et al.* confirmed (unpublished observations) that over 80% of the subjects who subsequently developed Type 1 diabetes were anti-GAD positive several year prior to the clinical onset of the disease. Type 1 diabetes has attributes consistent with it being an autoimmune disease, although there are some patients with Type 1 diabetes with insulin deficiency from other causes. Observations based on various sources of patients indicate that over 70% of newly diagnosed Type 1 diabetes subjects have high titre of anti-GAD and other features consistent with autoimmunity including ICI and antibodies to insulin. Apart from these features, the autoimmune process evolves to total islet beta-cell destruction since Type 1 diabetes in characterized by absolute insulin deficiency and life long insulin-dependency. Although hyperinsulinaemia is a characteristic of Type 2 diabetes, there are cases of Type 2 diabetes with genuine insulin deficiency, many are in non-obese category with a beta-cell secretary defect whereas a proportion, perhaps 10-15% are in transition to Type 1 diabetes. This subgroup has distinctive immunological and metabolic features that distinguish its members from those with Type 2 diabetes. These cases could be 'latent Type 1 diabetes' as judged by persistent ICA, progressive loss of beta-cells and high frequency of thyogastic autoimmunity. This group has special implication for Asian population where Type 1 diabetes in childhood is rare. It seems while yoga can definitely provide a better metabolic management of Type 2 diabetics, it has potential to protect against the development of 'latent' Type 1 diabetes.

References

1. World Health Organization, Expert Committee on Diabetes Mellitus: Technical Report Series 646, Geneva: WHO.
2. National Diabetes Data Group: Classification and diagnosis of diabetes mellitus and other categories of glucose intolerance. Diabetes 1979; 28:1039-1067.

Study of Vital Capacity of Lungs of Allergy–Asthma Patients After One Year Yoga Training

B.K. Bandre

Introduction

The Indian system of yoga philosophy has many fixed observances or binding which must be observed by student of yoga. This fact effects on those who want to get benefits from yoga practices. In this way yoga philosophy become applied yogic science.

With many studies, it is proved that yoga is helpful for the treatment of allergy and asthma. But the short term studies all over the world were proved the short term control on the above problem and methods used in the treatment were very much clumsy, lengthy and difficult to learn by a layman. It is found that these regular doing practices were very little helpful to the patients.

A very short term practice of 7 days of nonconventional therapy like Kunjal, Jalneti, Vastra Dhauti, Bhastrika and few asanas and kapalbhati as the therapeutic procedure for the treatment of allergy and asthma has been reported by several authors. The classical work conducted by Dr. Nagarathna and Nagendra have shown significant improvement in many patients under going yoga training. While they are in Vivekananda Ashrama. The subjective improvement in most of the patients occurred due to case in breathing with decreased air way resistance for some time during the day after yogic treatment.

Allergy and its chronic condition is asthma, these are constitutional disorder and has a psychosomatic basis. Imbalance in structure of the patient is a major cause for the problem. Body structure is mainly effected by life style of living, work and sleeping positions. These many contribute to possible decrease in blood flow towards the airways and organs involved in respiratory system.

Methods

The study was conducted on thirty five diagnosed cases of allergy and asthma with age range of 16 to 60 years. Few of them were effected by allergy only and were facing the difficulties in breathing. Most of them were in remission phase of asthma. These patients were treated by the local allergy specialists clinic, chest clinic and M.Y. hospital of Indore. The diagnosis was based on paroxysms of dysponea, wheezing and cough. They were treated for long time but unable to cure their problems. They reported to Indore school of yoga for yogic treatment. Most of them found the known practices of yoga *i.e.,* Jalneti, Kinjal, Dharti etc. were done by them. But they reported the partial benefits till they have done these practices.

Training in Yoga

Before starting yoga training at Indore school of yoga, they were instructed to sit erect while working, writing, reading, watching the T.V. and sleeping without the pillows at night. They were asked to sleep in "Shavasana" throughout the night. They were tested for lung capacity with the help of Peak Flow Meter (Deep breathing test of White Brothers). The average reading was 250 4 min. All the thirty five patients received thirty minutes yoga training. These consisted of Brahmamudra, Kandha sanchalana (Swami Janardhana), Marjari asana, Ushtrasana, Shashkasana Vakrasana, Mtysasana, Dhanurasana or Bhujangasana, Paschatya Pranayama of Swami Shivanand (Rishikesh), Uttan padasana and Shavasana.

After shavasana, Nadishodhan pranayama and three strocks of Bhastrika were given to the patients. Also lectures on the posture of body, cause to create to hyper sensitivity of nose and effect of wrong posture on the lung were given to them. Half an hour morning training for 7 day was enough to understand these above practices. After that they were doing their routine work in the same environmental condition and mental, physical work as they were having before. Specific diet control was not observed by them but the foods increase the allergy were stopped. The patients were asked to continue their medicine for few days and advised to record the change in drug reducing dosages. These patients were asked to visit the Yoga School every after one month for lung capacity test by peak flow meter. Through out the twelve months, their lungs capacity and condition of their health were recorded.

End of the six month the lungs average capacity value was 350 4 min. in all the patients. The results closely indicated the increased in tidal volume of the lungs by way of stretch and relaxation of voluntary inspiratory and expiratory muscles. After one year the average test value of 500 4 min; patients were free from attacks of asthma and allergy.

Discussion

Although the life style and correction in postures of sleeping and sitting were difficult to some patients for some time. To sleep in "Shavasana" without the pillow indicates normal parasympathetic and sympathetic function in asthma patients. Their nostrils and airways were clear in the morning. Before the yogic training and wrong posture, they were unable to breath from 4 a.m. onwards.

The link between autonomic and pulmonary function in patients after Yoga training have shown a strong association. End of the year all the patients stopped their medicine completely with profound elevation of symptoms and feeling of well being. Shavasan during the whole period of night facilitated by bio feed back have also shown reduction in airway resistance. Sleeping without pillow through out night reduced the size of sinues and hypersensitivity.

Application of Bandha on Psychosomatic and Psychiatric Disorders

D.N. Rai

Bandha in most modern Yogic literature is defined simply as 'Lock'. The Bandha group consists of Moola bandha Uddiyana bandha and Jalandhara bandha. The fourth Mahabandha is a combination of these three. Bandhas involve the contraction or squeezing of muscles. As there are three bandhas, there are three main muscle groups involved; perennial muscles, abdominal muscles and cervical (neck) muscles, contraction of these muscles affects the nervous, circulatory, respiratory endocrine and energy system.

Moola bandha stimulates both the sensory motor and the autonomic nervous systems in the pelvic region. When moola bandha is performed, pelvic stimulation activates parasympathetic fibers emerging from the pelvic spinal cord. Parasympathetic fibers emerge from the cervical (neck) and sacral (pelvic) areas only, while sympathetic before emerge from the thoracic (upper back) and lumbar (Lower back) areas. The performance of bandhas has been experimentally shown to enforce all Parasympathetic activities in the body which includes a decrease of heart rate, respiration and blood pressure and a general sense of rest and relaxation.

The Sanskrit word Moola means "root", firmly fixed, basis the foot, lowest part or bottom, foundation etc. Bandha means

"Lock restrain", "shut or close". Together the moola and bandha refer to the contraction of mooladhara chakra.

Moola bandha is known as the "Perineal lock" contraction of the muscles around the perineal body in the male and the cervix in the female. The physical contraction of the perineum has the beneficial effects of maintaining hormonal balance and stimulating and regulating the nervous that enervate the lower pelvic region, there by regulating all the internal organs.

Uddiyana bandha compresses the digestive organs, *adrenal gland,* kidneys and most important the *solar plexus uddiyana bandha* tones the *sympathetic nervous system,* encouraging it to work more efficiently, it also enables us to gain control over the sympathetic system so that it does not function in inappropriate situations. This avoiding the effects of stress and anxiety in Psychosomatic disease.

Jalandhara bandha stretches the neck, pulling the spinal cord and thus the brain. This has subtle effects on the pituitary and pineal glands while the forward flexion affects the *thyroid, parathyroid* and *thymus glands,* Jalandhara bandha also compresses the carotid sinuses, which help in lowering the blood pressure. By reducing sympathetic tone, one achieves a sense of rest, relaxation and general well being.

Moola bandha is an important tool in the treatment of physical disease of the *lower abdomen, digestive ailments* and *sexual disorders.* Moola bandha has the immediate effect of creating a deep sense of *mental relaxation therapy* relieving most mental and Psychosomatic disorders. Which are the direct or indirect effect of stress tension and anxiety.

As a mental relaxant, moola bandhas has been found extremely useful in the treatment of such mental disorders as *depression, nervous, phobia, hysteria* and mania. Moola bandha also helps to release the brahma growth (Psychic knot at mooladhara chakra) allowing the prana to flow up sushumna nadi.

Technique

Regarding the techniques and benefits of moola bandhas. In

chapter 9 of the **Health Yoga Pradipika** its states. "Press the heel against the perineum and contract it firmly. Draw the apana upwards. This is known as mool bandha."

The Gheranda Samhita States

"Press with the heel of the left foot the region between the anus and the scrotum and contract the rectum, carefully press the intestines behind the navel on the spine, and put the right heel on the organ of generation or pubes. This is called moola bandha, destroyer of decay." (GS. 3:14-17)

The Siva Samhita States

"Pressing well the anus with the heel, forcibly draw apana vayu slowly by precise. This is described as moola bandha, destroyer of decay and death. (S.S. 4:41-44)

Moola bandha is referred to in several of the Upanishads according to Yoga Tattva, Shandilya, Yoga Chudamani, and Yoga-Shikha Upanishads, the perfection of moola bandhas brings about the union of prana and apana. When they are joined together the union of Nada and Bindu can also take place. With this many Siddhis (Psychic abilities) are achieved. In the Dhyanabindu and Shandilya Upanishads it is also stated that he, who perfects moola bandha regains his youthful vitality and is victor over old age and death.

Moola bandha is also widely mentioned in modern yogic Indian and western literature.

Many translations of Hatha yoga texts describe moola bandha as pressing the heal against the perineum and contracting the Anus. The practice of moola bandha reactivates the areas in the brain controlling this region of the body, bringing the neuronal circuits responsible for its control into the sphere of consciousness.

Benefits

1. Psychotherapeutic Benefits

Moola bandha and bandhas in general are a powerful means of relaxing the body and mind. They relax the mental tenseness that we see in various personalities as phobia, *mania, hysteria,* and *anxiety.* Even schizophrenia and other psychoses are amenable to mool bandha if they are caught in their early stages and the personality has been previously stable.

Mool bandha increases the activity of the *parasympathetic nervous system, lowering the breathing* rate, heart rate, *blood pressure* and *stabilizing* the brain waves. The whole endocrine system is rebalanced. Which leads to stabilization and equilibrium of the personality.

2. Medical Benefits

Female: Moola bandha may be used to alleviate *dysmenorrhea* (painful menstruation *i.e.*) and *amenorrhea* (absence of period) moola bandha has also proved useful in child birth. A pregnant women may continue to practices right up to the time of labour in order or maintain elasticity in the vaginal muscles, aiding in painless delivery.

Moola bandha is also excellent for treating *prolapse, leucorrhoea* and *urinary (stress) incontinence.*

Male: Moola bandha alleviates *spermatorrhoea* (leakage of semen). Helps prevent inguinal hernia and controls testosterone secretion and sperm formation, pansies passions. Which influences coronary behaviour.

The practice of Moola bandha allows for a smooth Metamorphosis at menopause time by rebalancing hormonal changes, preventing such unpleasant symptoms as lethargy, *irritability, depression, high blood pressure* and giddiness. Thus moola bandha will ensure continuity of a healths, fulfilling life.

3. Benefits in Sexual Problems

Moola bandha is both a means to attain sexual control brahmacharya, and to alleviate a multitude of sexual problems. Moola bandha increases vitality. For this reason is extremely useful in treatment of many sexual problems of an inhibitory nature such as *impotance, fear of sexual expression and under performance etc.* The successful practice of moola bandha in these cases re-establishes *normal healthy sexual relations.* Thereby enhancing or recreating harmony in the total marital relationship.

Moola bandha also increases *sexual retention* power. The implications of this further magnify the possibility of retrieving the threads of a marital relationship threatened with extraction by the sexual dissatisfaction of one or both of its partners. With an increases in sexual retentiveness sexual relations become more satisfying and fulfilling.

Through the practice of moola bandha sexual relationship with tend to be more enjoyable and spiritually more meaningful. For by realizing the true nature of the primal energy residing in moola bandha. Your sexual partner becomes as one of the gods and the sexual act a symbolic expression of the union of Shiva and Shakti.

References

1. Gopal K.S. & Lakshmanan S., "Some observation on Hatha Yoga Bandhas: an Anatomical Study" Ind. J. Med. Sc. 26:9:1972.
2. Narayanananda, Swami, "The Primal Power of man; Prasad & Company, Rishikesh, India, 1960.
3. Rosenberg J.L., "Total organism", Random House Mc. U.S.A., 1975.
4. Satyananda, Swami, Tantra of Kundalini Yoga, Bihar School of Yoga, Munger, India, 1972.
5. Satyananda, Swami, Meditation from the tantras, Bihar School of Yoga, Munger, 1977.
6. Sivanand, Swami, "Science of Yoga". Vol. 4, Divine Life Society, Rishikesh, 1971.

Skin Care and Cure by Yoga and Neem

Rajesh Shukla

Neem is a religious, socio economical and environmental indicator plant since thousands of years. Neem is known as "Yauvana" "Wondercure" "Sarva Roganiwariri" tree proved by Saints & Yogis. Hindu believe Neem to be the royal child of mother nature.

In our Indian system of treatments like Unani, Prakratik, Tantra Mantra, Yoga are vigorously used in Ayurveda. It is also known that Neem plant is special gift for mankind. It is mentioned in ancient texts for Neem.

This plant is used for different cures in body from head upto skin.

Clinical Trial Report of Neem with Adjurant Yoga too on Psoriasis Patients

Aims and Object

To Evaluate Clinical Efficacy of Neem.

Trials Carried Out at

Government Ayurveda Dispensary, Makronia, Sagar (M.P.) on O.P.D. Patients with Panch Karma & Yoga.

Introduction

Neem leaves and Barks are used as extract for Swedan and Local application in the patients, of PSORIASIS and other skin disorders. Pre Clinical history & other assessments are done before and after therapy and results were noted.

Materials and Methods

52 Patients who visited the hospital room form December 1993 to January 1.1.97 were taken for the following clinical trails:

1. Tab Dermina 2. Syrup Hepoliv 3. Syrup Dermina (Upkaran Pharmaceuticals, Bhopal)
2. Panch Tiktaghrit
3. Chalmogra Oil–Somraji Oil, Jatyadi Oil.
4. Neem–1. Leaves for Swedan
   2. Bark for Kwath.
5. Yoga–Asanas are Conducted During Treatment.

Dietetics

Diet is taken with low salt, fat, light masalas, less rice, urad, channa, cooked dals, leafy vegetables. Salads, milk, roated meat, small fish, fruit, Salads. (No Banana, Apple, Orange) No bringle bhindi, pear, gram, groundnut, etc. cabbage, raddish, carrots are to be consumed more. Honey is also given.

Exercises

(1) Morning and evening fresh air walk.

(2) Bath with Neem Leaves boiled water.

(3) Laughing & Pranayam.

(4) Psoriasis patients are found under Stress and Strain. They are suggested to under go "Shavasan & Surya Namaskar" and they get relief after these exercises.

The patients are clinically assessed after one year of regular treatment.

Observations

We found remarkable improvements in the patients at the beginning of the treatment. In few of patients symptoms increased. Then gradually they improved by disappearing of new scars. Itching, irritation bowl habits also improved. Stressed patients were seen with smily look.

None of the patient dropped out of the treatment. They took regular treatments. Swedan by Neem leaves and Snehan by Chalmogra oil has given dramatic changes in skin. When patients have more than 60% changes over skin. Somraji oil was used at bed time.

After 80% improvement and also disappearance of Scars from Skin Jatyadi+Chandan Oil is applied. Skin became smooth and shining Dermina, Hepoliv+Panchtikta Ghrita (For Abhyantara Snehan) was also found very effective.

Conclusions

Dermina, Hepoliv, Panchtikta Ghrit, Neem+other oils are found very effective treatment for Psoriasis. With Control of Dietetics, excercises Asanas and routine habits. These drugs with Neem changes the whole skin activities and gives absolute cure for the endurable disease. In the prognosis on this disease is known that nomoderate or effective repairs.

References

1. Ayurveda Sar Sangrah.
2. Bhav Prakash.
3. Ras Tantra Sar Sanghrah.
4. Dravyagun Vigyan.
5. Sidhamala.
6. Bhaishaj Karma Sidhi.

Table 1

Clinical Trail Report of Neem with Therapeutic Ayurvedic Medicines Recovery after One Month

S. No.	Observations of Pt. Age Wide	Total	Effective	Moderate	Less	Nil	Male	Female	Remarks
01	One Year	15	10	-	5	-	11	4	
02	Five Year	10	-	5	3	2	6	4	
03	Eight Year	5	-	1	2	2	2	3	
04	Ten Year	7	1	3	2	1	5	2	
05	Twenty to Sixty Year	15	6	8	1	-	10	3	

Table 2

Recovery after Two to Six months

S. No.	*Observations of Pt. Age Wide*	*Total*	*Effective*	*Moderate*	*Less*	*Nil*	*Male*	*Female*	*Remarks*
01	One Year	15	14	1	-	-	11	4	
02	Five Year	10	3	1	1	5	6	4	
03	Eight Year	5	1	1	2	-	2	3	
04	Ten Year	7	3	1	1	2	5	2	
05	Twenty to Sixty Year	15	8	6	1	-	10	5	

–Dr. Rajesh Shukla
Sagar (M.P.)

Stress and Its Management

S. Singh & P.D. Mishra

In contemporary society, because of multiplicity of factors and forces, there is a lot of pressure of varied kinds on people, especially in terms of demand for fulfilment of evergrowing needs, particularly due to a availability of goods and services of numerous types made possible by rapid pace of development in the field of science and technology which was radically transform the communication system and reduced the entire world community into a global village. These pressures adversely tell upon nerves of people and lead to creation of varied kind of psycho-somatic disorders. Ever-increasing tempo of life has made it difficult for people to cope up with the new kinds of demands in the fast changing situations and force them to live under constant worry, anxiety and tension to the extent that relaxation of nerves up to the desired level does not become possible even after taking tranquilisers.

There are limits to tolerance of pressure, particularly the accumulated one, by both body and mind. Since every situation characterized by pressure creates an additional burden on the physical and mental capacities of people, varied kinds of psycho-physiological disturbances are created when the pressure created by situational demands exceeds the tolerance limits. In the past when the need of the people were limited and situations were relatively more simple, people could easily withstand the pressure of situation's in which they were place but now when even the sky is not the limit of the evergrowing list of demands which go on exerting accumulated pressures, human beings in contemporary society find it difficult to adapt to and adjust with them with the result that a lot of stress and strain is experienced by them which get manifested in different types of physical and mental ailments–many of them are of such types whose even name were not known to the mankind in the available history of medical systems of varied kinds.

I. Meaning and Definition

Broadly speaking, the term stress refers to a typical condition of mental of emotional disquiet. It is a non-specific response of a the body to any demand made on it. Stress is the tension and pressure that results when an individual views a situation presenting a demand that threatens to his or her capability or resources. Here we define stress as a person's adaptive response to stimulus that places excessive psychological or physical demands on him or her.[1]

It is the state of an organism where he perceives that his well-being is endangered and that he must divert all his energies to its protection.[2,3] We should not consider stress as imposed upon the organism, but as its response to internal or external processes which react these threshold levels that strain its physical and psychological integrative capacities close to or beyond their limits.[4] Stress is felt when one neither fights nor flights but remains a silent spectator and actor to the present stimuli. It refers to any such characteristics of the environment which poses a threat to the individual.

The stress was first used in a manner relevant for social sciences when the endocrinologist Hans Selye defined stress as the state manifested by a specific syndrome which consists of all the non-specifically induced changes within a biological system. Selye postulated a General Adaptation Syndrome (GAS) of somatic symptoms produced by non-specific stress. He postulated three stages in the GAS.[5]

1. The alarm reaction–In an initial shock stage resistance of the body is lowered followed by countershock during which the individual's defense mechanism become active.

2. Resistance stage–It is an stage of maximum adaptation and successful return to equilibrium.
3. Exhaustion–It is a stage when adaptive mechanism collapse. This stage comes when the stress prolongs.

Thus stress may be defined as a person's adaptive response to a stimulus that places excessive psychological or physical demands on that person. It is the pressure experienced by a person perceiving a stimulus in the environment which generates additional demands and disrupt the physical and mental functioning of the entire personality system. What actually happens is that any stimulus perceived by a person stimulates the nervous system which activates pituitary and adrenal glands leading to the secreation of various types of hormones which, when allowed to accumulate, produce various types of toxins and bring about innumberable changes in the body chemistry. In any situation in which new kinds of stimuli are perceived or the familiar stimuli in the modified forms are identified, a situation of fight-flight or freeze–the three kinds of possible responses–develop, and it is particularly in the situation of 'freeze' type of response that a lot of stress is experienced because the secreted hormones are not utilized.

II. Factors Responsible for Stress

A multiplicity of factors are responsible for creation of stress; and these can be broadly categorized into three groups:

1. Personality stressors,
2. Organizational stressors,
3. Environmental stressors.

Personality stressors include personality type perception, past experiences, attitudes, beliefs and value system, emotions and feelings, etc. In the category of organizational stressors can be included the demands relating to task to be performed and role to be played including ambiguity and conflict that may exist in them, organizational structure, organizational culture, pace of organizational change, rapidity of change in job, frequency of transfer opportunity for promotion, possibility of demotion quantum of work load, working conditions, conditions of work, particularly the availability of incentives, inter-personal demands of organization in terms of its development, type of leadership, opportunity for communication and participation, nature of interpersonal relationship, job security, nature of job in terms of involvement of new challenges, degree of inherent fear of failure in job mainly because of uncertainty with regard to successful job performance, long working hours without proper rest pauses, politicking, devolution of responsibility without corresponding authority and accountability, conflicting orders and demands from superiors, over expectations and unrealistic expectations of subordinates, conflict between task requirement and personal accomplishment, degree of prevailing lethargy and idleness on the part of employees, approach adopted by employees and their organizations–problem creating or problem shooting, unreasonable and undue demands of employees and their organizations, conflict between organizational and societal values, opportunities for career growth and development, availability of supportive services like guidance, counselling, help, especially in problem situations, etc. Environmental factors are innumberable but important among them are spiraling prices of commodities, deteriorating law and order situation, non-availability of adequate creative opportunities for utilization of surplus time, particularly in old age after retirement, uncertainties in all walks of life–economic, technological, political, educational, cultural and social; new kinds of demands and pressures, growing complexity of family problems, conflict, tension, unhygenic conditions not only in physical environment but also in socio-economic contexts immoral conditions, etc.

III. Consequences of Stress

There are a number of consequences of stress which may be broadly classified into two categories:

1. Positive consequences (Eustress)
2. Negative consequences (Distress)

Some kind of stress is essential for all kinds of actions without which any goal can not be successfully achieved. But the distress, particularly when it is in the accumulated form, is disastrous leading to several kinds of benefit consequences for the persons affected by it, for the family in which the person lives, for the organization in which the person works, and for the entire community and society at large to which he belongs. Harmful consequences for the person are reflected in varied kinds of disorders relating to different dimensions of health–the physical dimension, the mental dimension, the social dimension and the spiritual dimension. It is noteworthy here that the integrated concept of health necessarily implies that a person should be healthy not only in terms of absence of any kind of physical ailment but also in terms of the non-existence of any type of mental disorder, social malfunctioning and spiritual degeneration. In the context of family stress in the long run creates situation of family tension, family conflict, family disorganization and sometimes family disintegration. Baneful consequences of stress for organization are manifested in the non-achievement of organizational goals, creation of strained relations, and inability of the organization to fulfil even genuine needs of its employees and to solve even the most demanding problems. Community to which the person under stress belongs also ultimately suffers because the kind of social participation required for expected contribution to various programmes of development does not become available.

It has been proved by numerous studies that the living under continuous average stress leads to varied kinds of psycho-somatic disturbances. There are: Mental illness maladaptive behaviour physical diseases,[6,7,8] violent behaviour and habits of alcoholism and drug addiction.[9,10,11]

IV. Management of Stress

Stress management requires multidimental approach attacking it from all possible different corners. Various measures that may be adopted to manage stress may be classified under the following categories:

1. Change in personality structure
2. Organisational change and development
3. Environmental modification

Since it is an individual who is the victim of stress, changes in the personality structure are of utmost importance. Creation of right kind of attitudes and value system such that the person successfully cope up with the new situations or the old situations in their modified forms without experiencing any tension, anxiety or pressure.

The following technique are immensely helpful in controlling the stress, minimizing its physiological harmful effects and enhancing the immunity system of the body:

1. Hydrotherapeutic measures
2. Breathing exercises
3. Relaxative pestures
4. Meditation
5. Diet control

1. Hydrotherapeutic Measures

Purification of body is essential for the normal functioning. In naturopathy and yoga, purification in a special form of therapy employed for the elimination of waste products from the body. During stress, the rate of waste–production increases many times and if it is not bring out from the body it may cause may diseases, water therapy is the most appropriate therapy for purifying the body. These techniques are:

(i) ***Water sniffing :*** Water sniffing affects the circulatory system, respiratory system and nervous system directly and other systems indirectly. Lukewarm water dilates the capillaries of the nasal cavity, causing more blood to the areas of lower and upper brain. As a reactionary effect, the brains activities are first stimulated later an depressed for sometime. This has soothing effect on thinking process. Nerve fibres of parasympathetic are stimulated with the result one feels relaxation and happiness.

(ii) ***Stomach wash :*** Stomach is the main centre for metabolic activities. Timely cleansing of stomach is essential for the normal functioning of the body and mind. Drinking lukewarm water and vomiting it out helps in the dilation of

blood vessel, of the esophagies and stomach, provides extra nutrition to the abdominal muscles and increases peristalsis. The process puts more weight on heart and therefore it should not be practised by heart patients.

(iii) ***Colon cleansing*** : Colon is that part of GIT where excreta is accumulated and its timely cleansing is essential. To cleanse the colon enema is used. The lukewarm water removes the excreta, cleanse the colon, stimulates the muscles and improves the blood circulation. This helps in increasing appetite and mental peace.

(iv) ***Cold bath*** : Cold bath is a physiological tonic and has the advantage over medicinal tonics of all sorts. If awakens nerves activities without the imposition of any extra burden upon any vital organ. It makes impression upon the skin with its vast network of sensory, metor sympathatic, vasometer and thermic nerves. If activities every nerve centres, every sympathetic ganglion, every sensory and meter filament in the entire body to heightened life and activity.

(v) ***Coldfoot bath*** : The most important effects can be seen in vasometer and other reflex effects set up in the pelvic viscera causing contraction of the vessels and muscles of the genital organs. The effects can be seen on sympathetic and parasympathetic systems. Sympathetic nerve centres get soothing effect and their stimulation is regulated. Blood circulation in the internal organ increases. Brain gets tonic due to reflex effects. Respiratory mechanism is brought under control and depth of breathing increases. Due to all these reflex actions, the tensions in the muscles and nerves are reduced and one feels calm and peace.

(vi) ***Cold hip bath*** : In the cold hip bath, an impression is made upon the cutaneous areas which are reflexly connected with the various organs of the body. If produces profound effect on the activities of the skin, cutaneous vessels and nerves. Tonic effect are seen on colon, kindneys, stomach and urinary system.

(vii) ***Cold spiral bath*** : Spine is the base of all physical and mental activities. Cold spinal bath effects all the organs of the body through making impression on sympathetic and parasympathetic nerve fibres which mainly originate from the spine. The over stimulation of sympathetic nerve fibres are brought under control by stimulating retrogate fibres.

2. Breathing exercises

Breathing means living and *vice-versa* oxygen is indispensable for life. Every living tissue and cell requires a constant supply of energy to live. To be alive means to undergo certain bio-chemical process which takes place by the energy. The energy is restored in the molecules of food substances. It is released through oxidation. But oxidation can not take place without oxygen. Therefore every cell must get sufficient oxygen which does not happen in the agitated and stressed mind. Pranayam is a specialized technique to control the breathing and provide the opportunity to reach oxygen in the very cell of the body. During stress, breathing system is disturbed and shallow breathing occurs. This may cause various physical diseases, *i.e.,* tuberculosis, asthma, headache etc. In Pranayama, all the muscles are relaxed, contracting only respiratory muscles in the acts of Puraka and Recbaka. This helps to give the body and mind complete rest and to eliminate tension from the mind.

3. Relaxative Postures

The aim of relaxation is the release of tensions working at the level of muscles and nerves. Tensions are the result of external stresses or continuous internal thought processes. Tense muscles and nerves obstruct the blood flow and easily get exhausted. Tensed nerves disintegrate the harmony of the body.

Shavasana, Shashankasana and Makarasana are three postures or asanas for maximum relaxation of the body and mind.

(*i*) ***Shavasana*** : It provides the most natural position of the body. Anatomically no position can be better than this for the complete relaxation. Horizontal position of the body on ground helps in the normal flow of blood. No system of body is required to work against the gravity. No extra energy is required to any system of the body, therefore metabolic rates come down. Even the blood pressure and heart rate reduced to minimise because there is no need of force to circulate the blood. The O_2 requirement is reduced, therefore less production of CO_2. The intensity of stress impulses is minimised and sympathetic over-activities are slowed down. It helps in falling of arterial blood pressure, slowing pulse rate and muscles tone.

(ii) ***Shashankasana*** : Shashank means moon. This posture provides the benefits of moon. It is very effective in cooling down the aggressive tendencies and tenseful conditions. Because the first posture is of Vajrasana, so it gives all benefits of Vajrasana also.

(iii) ***Makarasana*** : It helps in relieving fatigue and tension both physical and mental level and provides extra psychic energy for dealing a net set of problems.

4. Meditation

Meditation is a yogic technique which has recently become popular all over the world. There have been hundreds of researches on psycho-physical responses during and after meditation and its therapeutic uses. Regular practice of meditation helps infalling down the cholestrol level and plasma cortisal level which is considered as an important bio-chemical indicator of stress.

5. Diet Control

Diet occupies a dominant place in the naturopathy and yoga practice. It is said that 'as you eat, so you become'. This is because the kind and quality affects the physical as well as mental condition of the individual. Thus, the individual who does not take a proper diet and who does not have a proper understanding of the principles of eating, gradually begins to harm himself both physically and mentally. Vegetarian diet is the appropriate diet for stress releasing. In the diet, fruit, salad, leafy vegetables, green vegetables should be included. These items helps in energizing the whole organs of the body and cool down the mental stress.

In short, it can be concluded that the application of neturopathy and yoga brings about sound health and long life particularly with the help of various methods and techniques which give suppleness to the spine–our very life axis–by calming over-wrought nerves, by relaxing muscles, and by reviving organs and nervous centres. Development of the right kind of attitude towards life as cited below can be of immense help in getting rid of the unnecessary anxiety, tension and worry that all of us suffer from quite often.

But what is the use worrying? You are either going to live or die. If you live, there is no use to worry, if you die, you will either go to Heaven or Hell. If you go to Heaven, there is nothing to worry about. If you go to Hell, you will be so busy shaking hands with all your friends that you would not have time to worry.

References

1. Moorhead, Gregory and Griffin, Ricky W. : Organizational Behaviour, Managing people and organization, Jaico Publishing House, Bombay, 1994, p. 454.
2. Caplan, R.D., S. Cobb and J.R.P. French: "Relationships of cessation of smoking and Job Stress, Personality and Social Support" Journal of Applied Psychology, 1975, Vol. 60, p. 211-219.
3. Cofer, C.N. and Appley, M.H.: Motivation: Theory and Research Wiley, 1964, quoted by Marshall J. Cooper, C.L.: Executives under Pressure, The Mac Millan Ltd., 1979, p. 7.
4. Basowitz, H. Persky, H. Korchin S.J. and Grinker, R.R.: Anxiety and Stress, Mac Graw Hill Co., New York, 1955, quoted by Marshall, *Ibid.,* p. 7.
5. Selye, H.: The Stress of Life, McGraw Hills Comp. New York, 1956, quoted by Sharma, B.R., "Administrative Stress" IIPA, New Delhi, 1986, p. 3.
6. Eisentadt, S.: Modernization: Protest and Change, Engleword Cliffs, Prentice Hall, 1966; Wolfe and Goodell, H.: Stress and Disease, Charles C. Thomas, Springfield Ill, 1968; Jaco, E.: "Mental Illness in Response to Stress" in S. Levine and N. Scotch (ed.), Social Stress, Aldine Publishing Co., Chicago, 1970; and Toffler, A.: Future Shock, Random House, New York, 1970.

7. Eisentadt *op.cit.;* Spradly, J. and Phillips, M.: "Culture and Stress" American Anthropologist, 1972, p. 74.
8. Ogilvie, H.: The Tired Business, Charles C. Thomos, Springfield, Ill, 1964, and Wolfe and Goodwell *op.cit.*
9. Dodge, D. and Martin, W.: Social Stress and Chromic Illness Noitre Dame, 1970, and Coser, L.: Social Conflict and Theory of Social Change, British Journal of Sociology, 1957, Vol. 8.
10. Borg, M.: Conflict and Social Change, A. Publishing House, Minneapolis, 1971;

    Marlowe, L.: Social Psychiatry, Helbrook Press, Bostan, 1971.

Yoga–Its Therapeutic Utility as a Preventive Medicine

Rakesh Kumar

Yoga–the ancient cult of Indian heritage has become popular the world over during the past few decades. Not only as a health preserver and its promoter, but also on its way very much like a side effect or a bonus it helps in providing relief in many diseases which are resistant to conventional forms of therapy. Besides being free from the side effects commonly encountered in the drug therapy, yoga is a simple, safe, effective and highly economical form of adjunctive therapy. Therefore, though slowly but surely, it is being integrated into the mainstream of modern medicine.

Yoga, evolved as a system for liberation, with its ultimate goal of attaining an orgasmic state of trance, for a prolonged period, grants one with a bonus comprised of freedom from disease, healthy and long life, *i.e.* an objective than can be achieved without the use of drugs. In other words, yoga can play a significant role as preventive medicine in the modern times.

To made an easy understanding, let us discuss the concept of health, disease and preventive medicine.

Concept of Health in Yoga

In Hindi, health is translated as 'Swasthya', which is derived from the word swasth. It is composed of two words; swah tha, 'swah' means its own and 'tha' means site. In this way, swasthya means that state of human body in which all the bodily elements including doshas, dhatus, agnis, malas etc. (in modern sciences these can be considered as all bodily organs like heart, brain, glands, lungs, kidneys etc.) functions at their own site in the integrated and co-ordinative manner to provide a sense of well being at physical, mental, emotional and spiritual levels. Thus, Ayurveda in Susruta Samhita 51/44 states:

समदोष: समधातु समाग्निश्च मलक्रिय:।
प्रसन्न आत्मेन्द्रिय मन: स्वस्थ इत्यभिधीयते।।

A body is said to be healthy, when all the doshas, agnis, dhatus and mala's functioning is in homeostatic state to provide a sense of well being to mind, sense-organs and individual consciousness.

Concept of Disease in Yoga

The word 'disease' is composed of dis+ease. 'Dis' is prefix and used in negative sense. 'Ease' means comfort. That means the state of uneasiness of body is called disease.

In Hindi, disease is known as Vyadhi; *i.e.,* Vi+Adhi. 'Vi' is used in -ve sense and 'Adhi' is used for state of integration. That means the state of disintegration of the body is called Vyadhi or disease. In the light of concept of health, when the bodily elements including doshas, malas, agni, dhatus etc. do not function in co-ordinative and integrated way to provide a sense of discomfort or pain at physical, mental, emotional and spiritual levels, that state of body is said to be diseased.

Concept of Preventive Medicine

Generally, the word 'medicine' is used for a substance taken orally for a cure of disease. Actually, the literally meaning of medicine also includes 'art of healing'. That means any of the measures whether a substance taken orally or physical means including norms of diet, physio-therapy, natural means of Naturopathy, magnetotherapy, accupressure, accupuncture, yogic practices including Yamas and Niyamas, asnas, pranayama, mudras, meditation and other yogic norms for management of a disease, or cure of a disease/and maintenance of health etc. is called a medicine. Thus, medicine is not to be considered as a substance but also as a 'art of healing' with an aim of restoring health from a state of disease.

Yoga can play a significant role in the field of preventive medicine in modern times. As the drugs used for cure, have been becoming costlier as well as providing serious side effects, the people are giving serious thoughts for alternatives like magnetotherapy, accupressure, accupuncture, etc. There are some incurable diseases like AIDS, Cancer, Leukemia etc. for which the doctors, therapists, Govt. medias are stressing for preventive measures. Need of the hour is to popularize the preventive measures with the help of which common man would be able to maintain health and develop strong inherent defence mechanism to fight with internal/external offending agents of diseases. The brief account of various yogic means is hereby described to highlight the role of yoga as preventive medicine:

1. Role of Yamas and Niyamas : According to principles of yogic therapy, yamas and niyamas are the essential components to develop correct psychological attitude for the management of psychosomatic diseases like Asthma, Hypertension, Gastric acidity and ulcer, headache etc. Simple awareness of the norms of social and personal ethics for observance, help a patient to avoid further deterioration of the disease. Now all the medias are stressing for preventive measures for AIDS by avoiding excessive sex especially with partners other than wife, use of condoms, etc. Actually, the need of the hour is to provide the teaching of celibacy at school, college and university level. Correct meaning and principles of Brahamcharya for a family man are also to be stressed. The scientific values of -va and +ve emotions on the human body alongwith role of ethics (yamas and niyamas) in health and medicine are to be taught to college and university students.

2. Role of Satkarmas : In the yogic treatment, the purificatory processes have an important task for the management and prevention of the disease.

Neti is an important means to develop resistance against environmental offending factors like temperature, dust, pollengrains, humidity and other particles to prevent the respiratory disorder, for example, the neti in the evening by the labourers working at flour mills, cotton textiles mills, mines, dusty roads, harvesting grains in the fields, libraries etc. can wash out the inhaled particles and thereby preventing their decay and decomposition in nasal passage and pharynx for viral and bacterial infection. The use of neti helps also in development of resistance against seasonal change by using water of different temperature in neti lota during the period of change of season as it would increase the adaptability of inner lining of nasal passage for vaso-constriction and dilution in response to temperature variation of the environment.

Similarly, one can prevent digestive disorders by the use of shankhprakhshalana at the time of start of new season, basti once in a month, daily practice of nauli etc. In case of dyspepsia, the vaman dhoti/vyagrah dhoti will be useful to prevent intensity of digestive disorder. The regular practice of tratak and kapalbhati can be used to prevent the eye and respiratory disorders respectively.

3. Role of Asnas : Asnas play significant role in toning up the neuro-musculo-glandular system of the body to restore/maintain the vitality of bodily organs.

Asnas, as a preventive medicine, can be used for avoiding the causation of postural deformities like cervical spondylosis (by bhujang/dhanush/matsay/ustrasnas etc.) lordosis (hal/pawanmukta/paschimotanasna etc.).

Asnas can be used for release of physical stress resulted from day-to-day -ve emotions of the behavioural pattern. This will help to avoid psychosomatic or psychological disorders like hypertension, gastric acidity, depression, neurosis etc. The regular correct practice of asnas also help to prevent constipation, arthritis, asthma, diabetes, obesity etc.

4. Role of Pranayama : Pranayama has its important role in prevention of diseases. The various diseases caused by disturbed homeostatic state of autonomic nervous system like obesity, hypertension, hyperthyoiridism, diabetes, gastric acidity etc. can be prevented by nadishodhan pranayama, bhastrika pranayama etc. The imbalanced state of doshas caused in different seasons can be prevented by the practice ujjai, sitali, suryabhedan and bhastrika pranayamas. The intensity of psychosomatic ailments can be prevented by restoring the normal rhythmic breathing by the practice of pranayama.

5. Role of Meditative Practices : The regular practice of meditation by any of the various techniques, the inherent defence mechanism to fight with external physical, mental, emotional and environmental factors for causation of diseases can be developed. The meditation provides physical and mental resting pause to restore and revitalize the bodily organs for their normal functioning. Meditative practices have been widely used to counteract the day-to-day stress and strains of modern life. Therefore, the meditation can be used for prevention of psychological and psychosomatic disorders like depression, anxiety, nuercsis, hypertension, asthma, arthritis, angina etc.

6. Swarayogic and Dietary norms : Various norms of swara yoga and yoga dietetics also helps in prevention of diseases. Some important norms are:

1. The moderation of diet, intake of meals during surya swara, observance of sequence while taking food; *viz.* sweet articles taken firstly, sour and saline in middle and puncent and astrigent lastly; helps in digestion avoids causation of digestive disorders. Taking water after 1/2 to 3/4 hrs. of meals, avoiding sweet dishes at the end of meals, taking hot potency articles during chadra swara and cold potency articles in surya swara also prevents the causation of diseases in respect of digestive disorders, respiratory disorders etc.
2. Sleeping by keeping the head in the geographical south direction and lying on left side of the body helps to maintain health and prevents the causation of cardio-vascular ailments especially.
3. Taking bath during the surya swara also prevents the causation common cold, digestive disorders arthritis etc.
4. Avoiding the intake of betels during surya swara prevents the diseases of biles and pitta doshas like hypertension, acidity etc.

Yoga for the Improvement of Memory (Medhā Sanskār)

S.V. Vyavahare

Yoga–Very Useful Ancient Wisdom

People think that yoga means only few asanas, some pranayamas and dharna-dhyana only. But yoga has other practical applications too. Regular and proper yogic practices help solve many problems, concerning memory and concentration which majority of the students are facing every day.

Suicides in Japan

Taking inspiration from the news "number of the students committing suicides in Japan is increasing at alarming rate" a project named "MEDHA SANSKAR" was prepared and successfully implemented. "MEDHA" means memory and "SANSKAR" means "educating, training, polishing." So "MEDHA SANSKAR" means "training and polishing the memory."

Medha Sanskar

In ancient times, such medha sanskar was made on a boy of 8 years on the fourth day of "Upanayan Sanskar" (thread ceremony) by performing some rituals and chanting medha mantras. Very next day, the boy used to start for 12 year's learning at Guru's ashram. Since the printing press, books and schools nothing was existing, the boy, learning at Guru's ashram, was supposed to receive, register, retain, recollect and reproduce the knowledge imparted by Guru without any revision. So to have very sharp memory and one pointed concentration was need of the circumstances. That is why "Medha Sanskar" was performed under the name of "Medha Janana Prayoga" on the previous day of departure to Guru's ashram. This is, in short, the explanation why the project was named "MEDHA SANSKAR".

Educational Stress

Now coming back to the news of increase in the percentage of suicides being committed by students of the schools and colleges of Japan, attentions is drawn to the news published in "The Sunday Times" dated 8th Oct. 1995 about the Indian counterpart. The news says "Hundreds of students in the Bombay metropolis who are under 18 are undergoing psychiatric treatment. Psychiatrists attribute this disturbing trends to stress created by competitive education among other factors."

"Most of these children study in tenth or twelfth standard" says the head of KEM Hospital, Bombay, Psychiatry Department, Dr. Shubhangi Parkar, who claims that almost 75 percent of these children and adolescent patients have psychological problems pertaining to educational stress."

Aggressive Students

Students under stress become aggressive or show withdrawal symptoms. They have night mares, weight loss, talk in their sleep or crumble under severe academic strain.

Frustrated Students Commit Suicide

Some frustrated students go to extremity and end their life by committing suicide. According to figures available with the National Crime Records Bureau of India (NCRB), 11.2 per cent of approximately 85,000 suicide victims in the country in 1993 were children. A Majority of these cases were related to educational stress. The NCRB report, which describes the trend as a "matter of grave concern" recommends extensive studies on the issue, both in the governmental and nongovernmental spheres.

This action plan was already thought of by Yogacharya Shrikrishna Vyavahare of Thane (India) in 1985.

Yogic Solution

After carefully studying the various obstacles coming in the way of concentration and recollection, the yogic solutions were found out. The first "memory increasing class" was taken in 1985. Till such time, the book named "MEDHA SANSKAR" was published on 15th August 1993, 962 students were given proper guidance by conducting 9 such classes. After publication of the book such classes got impetus with the result that up to December 1996, 12,500 students took part in 65 Medha Sanskar Classes. Then the question arises "What are the obstacles coming in the way of concentration-reception-retention-recollection and reproduction, how to remove these obstacles with certain simple yogic practices, how the classes are conduct and with that result?" Now we will try to find out the answers one by one without going into much details.

Tremendous Potential Lying Unattended

Basically each and every students is having tremendous potential but for the proper guidance and deeper realisation it is lying unattended, unused. Not a single student wants to get plucked in the examination. Everybody wants to get through with flying colours. Why majority of them are not successful? Why many of them are suffering from educational stress and few of them commit suicide on getting failure?

Parental Expectations Precipitates Psychological Imbalance

Educationsits and doctors say "competitive curriculum does not trigger depression. However, when it is coupled with parental expectations, the indifference of the teachers and pressure from the peer groups, it certainly precipitates psychological imbalance in most students". In addition, students tend to become more and more fatalist then conatus, self-reliant.

Fatalism not Existing

In Yoga Vasistha, Vasistha tells Ram that fate as such is not existing at all. Fatalists are nothing but great fools. It is just to pin point his failure that man has created "FATE". If a man makes very honest and sincere efforts in a very right direction, he is bound to get anything under the sky.

Five Steps in Progression *(प्रयत्न पंचपदी)*

In the very begining of the "Medha Sanskar Varg (Class)" the golden thoughts of Sage Vasistha are explained to the students in a very simple language and light mood. Thus the background for rejecting the fatalism and accepting the challanges is prepared and on this sound foundation the whole programme is structured in the following five steps in progression.

(1) Concentration (केन्द्रीकरण)

Obstacles	*Solution*
(1) Unstable body posture	Stable body posture
(2) Stiff body posture	Relaxing body posture
(3) Incorrect body posture	Correct body posture
(4) Blocked vasal passage	Cleansing Kriya:
	(a) Shvasan Marg Shuddhi (with the nostril)
	(b) Kapalbhati (with two nostrials)

Now a days, concentration is not the problem, but concentration with relaxation is the problem. Unless the students are able to relax on physical and mental level, they will not have better concentration and if there be any, they will get headache.

(2) Reception (ग्रहण)

Ours is a multichannel receiving system of knowledge. We receive knowledge and information through five sense organs. Even though we are having quiet efficient sensory system, if the mind is wondering somewhere and not alert and attentive, even the simple knowledge is not received through any sense organ and further registered in the brain. Following are some of the obstacles coming in the way of receiving knowledge.

Obstacles	*Solution*
(1) Random/extrovert mind	Prana Dharana (Breath awareness)
(2) Speedy breathing	Slow/deep breathing
(3) Multiple subjects in the brain	Bhramari Pranayama
(4) Agitated/excited/upset mind	OM chanting.

(3) Retention (धारणा)

Brain is having tremendous capacity to retain knowledge that we are receiving throughout our life. We can store hundreds and thousands and lacs of various types of incidents in the memory. If we try to recollect all the stored knowledge at a time, we will either go mad or get confused. So we should be able to make the 'Switch On' for the required knowledge concerning the situation in hand and 'off' for the unwanted information registered in the brain. That is why it is very important to forget unwanted subjects and remember the wanted answers in our daily routine in general and examination in particular.

Why We Forget?

We very essily forget what is meaningless, useless and six disorganised. Similarly many a times, we forget simple thing due to fears, fobias, complexes, tensions, worries, fatigue, ill health, lack of rest or sleep, overexertion etc. Acute hunger or heavily loaded stomach also comes in the way of recollection.

(4) Recollection (Memory) (स्मरण)

Memory According to Ancient Indian Texts

According to Upanishadas, Patanjali's Yoga Sutras and Ayurveda, "smriti"-memory is one of the powers of the mind. If the mind is weak, memory is weak. If the mind is impure, the memory is also very poor. To make the mind and resultant memory pure, powerful and concentrated, OM chanting, Prayer, Mantra, Japa, devotional songs, some spiritual practices are necessary.

Memory–A Modern Concept

Is is very difficult to define memory and pinpoint the memory centre in the brain. Whether memory is in the form of chemical component or electrical activity or combination of both or something else is a matter of all round research. According to Dr. Cecil Lobe, Dr. Arthur C. Guyton memory is a part of nervous system.

Whether memory is a part of nervous system or one of powers of the mind, it is sure and certain that both (nervous system and mind) can be trained through proper Yogic practices.

Types of Memory

Mainly there are two types of memory (1) Short term memory and (2) Long term Memory. Short term memory is also called telephone memory, primary memory or immediate memory because it is a short lived memory. Such temporary memory is of no use to students from examination and career point of view. Now the question is how to convert short term memory into long term memory?

How to Make Short Term Memory Permanent

We can make the impressions permanent in the memory by

(1) Remaining alert at the time of learning.
(2) Making revision intermittently.
(3) Doing the proper classification.
(4) Understanding the subject with its meaning.
(5) Making short notes of the subject already understood.
(6) Arranging the study material properly.
(7) Remaining tension free.
(8) Keeping healthy-away from diseases and dosages.
(9) Relaxing the body and mind.
(10) Avoiding to become fatalist.
(11) Becoming self-reliant.
(12) Getting courage and confidence.
(13) Realizing the tremendous hidden potential.
(14) Doing systematic study without any fatigue.
(15) Removing the lethargy.

(16) Becoming active and alert.
(17) Avoiding excessive indulgence.
(18) Taking proper food and rest.

It is very easy to understand all the above items but they appear rather difficult to put into practice. But it is not so. Very few asanas, pranayamas, Kriyas, relaxation technique, OM chanting etc. help unearth our potential, remove negative thinking and bestow the required physical and mental power transforming the personality structure. More emphasis is given on practicals.

(5) Reproduction (प्रक्षेपण) (Transmission)

Students get very good marks in the examination only when they reproduce the subject in minimum words, with simple language writing to the point by observing the rules of grammer properly. This requires daily practice which gives courage, confidence and concentration, which help better recollection, and reproduction simultaneously.

Pilot Study

In order to evaluate the utility of Medha Sanskar classes and get the proper feed back, a questionnaire form was sent to 2500 students. 1889 students returned the forms duly filled in. Everybody liked the class and the course and found it very easy. The most important feature is that 97 percent emphatically said they would never become fatalist but would be compatus and self-reliant. This positive approach is very much encouraging. It shows a fundamental change in the thinking pattern of the students. So really speaking there is a total personality development under the name of memory development.

Further Research

Project for doing research is being prepared under the guidance of educationists, psychologists and yoga experts. It will be implemented in the next academic year (1996-97) results be published for the benefits of all. The research has already been started.

Therapeutic Role of Religion & Yogic Sciences in Mental Tension

K.K. Sharma

1. Introduction

"Health" is a state of complete well-being at physical, mental, social, moral and spiritual levels. Spiritual dimension of health as recognised by World Health Organisation recently has given new impetus to man's well-being and happiness. Fastly changing lifestyle of man in the midst of material pursuits, has put him under a great stress, strain, tension and mental imbalance. Since man degraded himself from the evolutionary process of high consciousness, he is destined to face new challenges in life. In this situation, "Religion" and "Yogic Sciences" play a vital role. The present paper is an attempt to draw our attention towards therapeutic role of religion and Yogic Sciences. It is highlighted that religion and yogic sciences including Sufism and mysticism, in the process, not only help to achieve new contours of spirituality but also possess a therapeutic and curative potential.

2. Present States of Man

Materialism has taken over our lives. At every moment we are confronted with choices without exercising an element of contentment. Repeatedly people are choosing the materialistic style of life. Where does this trend come from? Is it new? Is it modern? Does it come from Western Societies? Is it the effect of science? To my understanding, it is man's own creation. Man has given more importance to external material development in order to achieve comforts, happiness and peace. Consequent upon the same, it has taken man away from his real self and natural state of spirituality, that helps him to know his self, to make him complete human being and to know whether or not there is a God in heaven, there is certainly one within our self.

2.1 Effect of Materialism of Man

Modern advancements in science and technology have created new external stimuli. No doubt, they have a function as they increase our data banks and help us to grow. But too much sensory information numbs our thinking ability, thus the constant inflow does not let us listen to our self and does not give us time to assimilate the information.

Man is always under stress and strain in the midst of fast competitive society. The sustained state of stress leads to mental tension and hypertension. In technologically advanced and affluent societies, hypertension is reaching epidemic proportion. Even the third world countries are now having their share of persons suffering from hypertension. Moving from an agriculture based economy to highly congested and sophisticated economically, competitive zones, with poor housing and sanitation, impure water, adulterated food, chemical poisons from industries, every person, rich or poor is being affected of this dreaded disease.

2.2 Tension and Hypertension

As stated above, with more advancement at all fronts of materialistic life, man remains under a stressful environment. Stressful state of mind created by worry, anxiety, fear, insecurity, etc. for a larger duration leads to tension and hypertension. Following are the main causes which give rise to tension and hypertension.

- *(i)* A rich protein diet
- *(ii)* Regular use of alcohol
- *(iii)* Too much of smoking
- *(iv)* Little or no exercise

(v) Heavy atmospheric pollution
(vi) Too much pressure of work
(vii) High aspirations and ambitions
(viii) Aggressive behaviour

All these factors lead to an agitated life style, irregular habits, frayed nerves, inability to relax, insomnia, lack of faith due to lack of harmony in life, over individualistic attitude and so on.

Dr. S.R. Shah said, "High blood pressure" is a common symptom of hypertension. It damages various organs in the body namely, the brain, heart, kidneys, eyes, etc. Normal blood pressure reading is 120/80 mm/hg (120 systolic 80 diastolic). In persons living a long life, the pressure is usually on the lower side 100-110/60 mm/hg.

In most of the cases of hypertension, modern science cannot find an obvious cause. However, in some cases kidney diseases, endocrine gland disorders, etc., are responsible for hypertension. It has been found that age, heredity, too much salt intake, obesity, mental stress and smoking are the contributory factors.

3.0 Therapeutic Role of Religion, Mysticism and Yogic Sciences

Religion, Mysticism and Yogic Sciences have great potential to contribute to the positive health of human society in general and hypertensive patient in particular. Medical statistics state that over 80% of world's diseases are caused by the mind's stresses and tensions are the main factor involved.

Various religions and mysticism have been the long traditions practised by man over the ages for his spiritual development. Since spirituality is the essence of man's nature, religions and faiths of the world have had brought out a variety of philosophies, beliefs, practices and techniques to attain the same. The whole process was an attempt to realise best in man through a divine relationship with God or Cosmic Reality. In this regard, religion has been playing both a promotive and preventive role.

Distinctively Yogic Science especially Ashtanga Yoga has an additional role, that is, curative, as it encompasses human anatomy, physiology in its practice. This aspect has been dealt elsewhere in this paper.

3.1 Bases of Religion and Yogic Sciences

Both religion and yoga have common underlying assumption that man as an entity has three dimensions/levels of his existence:

(a) Physical (body)

(b) Mental (mind)

(c) Spiritual (spirit/soul/atman)

Man's development is considered in totality not in fragmentation since there is unity of purpose in human evolution which is the design of God or Cosmic Reality. A brief mention of three dimensions/levels of man's existence is made here for better understanding of the therapeutic role of religion and yoga.

(a) Physical Basis: Under physical dimension, we will have to understand human anatomy and physiology, that is, bones and their functions; blood–its composition, purity and function; cells, tissues, muscles, organs and systems-structure and functions; breathing–prana shakti (Bio-energy), types of prana, control and regulation of breath for elimination of toxins from the body; and physical environment–purity and cleanliness.

(b) Psychological Basis: Under psychological basis, we will have to understand the mind, and its functioning and related aspects. Some of the salient features are listed as under.

(i) Four states of mind–unconscious, sub-conscious, conscious and super-conscious.

(ii) Three gunas–sattvic, Rajsic and Tamsic.

(iii) Five Kosas–Annamaya Kosa, Pranamaya Kosa, Manomaya Kosa, Vijnanmaya Kosa, Anandamaya Kosa.

(iv) Five Klesas–Avidya (ignorance), Asmita (egoism) Raga (attachment), Dvesa (aversion) and Abhinives (desire to cling to life).

(v) Bhavas (feelings)–positive bhavas and negative bhavas.

(c) Philosophical Basis: Under philosophical basis, we refer to purpose of life, concept of man and his relation with nature, Atman (spirit/soul), God or Cosmic Reality and relationship of Atman with Paramatman.

3.2 Some Observations in Medical Sciences in relation to Stress and Therapy

(i) Nerve fibers (Naditantu) represent exceedingly fine tissues like those of the spider's threads and these connect all the nerve centres throughout the body like cobwebs. It is the movement of bioenergy within these nerves that sustains the living organism. In this regard any change or variation in Prana (Bioenergy) does affect man's health at different planes.

Therefore, recitation of holy or divine name (Mantra) or doing Japa or Naam Japa (in Sikhism) or keeping a Vision of God (in mysticism), or having purification of nervous system (Nadisuddhi) in Hath yoga, all accelerate the process of re-distribution of bioenergy in body. Even undertaking a holy work or virtuous task brings spiritual energy into the system. It acts as a therapy (curing physical and mental ailments).

(ii) Dr. S.M. Katrak says that mind is of paramount importance in the healing process as it is through the mind that we get motivated and motivation or arousal in state of mind is very much important for healing.

(iii) Mr. William Selvamurthy, Director, Defence Institute for Physiology and Allied Sciences (DIPAS) Delhi has observed the following in relation to stress management in his experiment on Effect of yoga Training for six months on 30 soldiers.

- Those in the yoga group, experienced reduced heart beat rate, lowered blood sugar level, higher skin temperature, slow breathing and increase in alpha index in EEG (present when the brain is quiet and calm).
- Yoga controls sympathetic activity. It keeps at low state which is under the control of part of the brain (at

the base) called hypothalamus. It regulates the release of stress hormones and is controlled by the limbic system in the brain, which in turn, is controlled by the cerebral cortex.

- During yogic practice, brain chemistry undergoes a change which further affects change in hypothalamus through the limbic system. This changed brain chemistry helps the person to remain calm and quiet during stress.
- In Yogic exercises, attention is needed to what one is doing. The role of concentration here is very significant that other exercises which are done mechanically. Concentration influences the brain which increases the synthesis of neurotransmitters like serotonin, dopomine and norepinephrine.
- Yoga cures stress–related diabetes and high blood pressure as it regulates hormones like adrenalin, noradrenalin and glucocorticoids (stress hormones) and also increases the synthesis of insulin.

(iv) Studies reveal that there is direct relationship between different moods and activity of immune cells, turning it up or down. Sleep and displays of emotions can prove to be healthy for the immune system while chronic stress, depression and over-anxiety are not. The brain and the immune system talk to one another that much is certain (Dasgupta, 1995).

(v) Dr. P. Mamtora (1995) says that a positive mental attitude is necessary both for the prevention and for the cure of arthritic conditions. In a happy person, the hormones secreted, boost the immune system and help to fight disease more effectively. With a positive attitude, a patient can reverse, develop and strengthen his immue system which can effectively correct the auto-immune responses.

Yoga and religion look at the individual in his totality at the physical, mental, emotional and spiritual levels. At the mental level, one must have faith and must learn art of relaxation. Naam Japa and Yogic techniques like Nispanda bhavna, Savasana and Dradhasana can appreciably bring down the level of stress.

Dr. P. Mamtora (1995) at the Yoga• Institute, Bombay teaches four qualities to keep positive frame of mind. They are–Maitri (Friendliness), Karuna (Compassion), Mudita (joy in the joy of others) and Upeksa (indifference to ups and downs). Besides this, practice is combined with "sattvic diet" taken every four hours.

(vi) Dr. P.K. Dave (1995) says stress causes spasm of muscle and this chronic state of spasm causes spinal pain. Yoga helps in lowering blood pressure and possibly induces better electroencephalographic changes and relaxes muscles to the state of normal functioning.

(vii) Hossaini Sayed Hashem (1995) psychotherapist from Iran observes the following:

- I realise that psychotherapy, psychoanalysis and psychopharmacology are not sufficient to cure psychiatrist patients. It is my feeling that something more should be added and I think spirituality is a means.
- For curing patients of having mental problems, there is need to study their experiences at different stages of growth and development–childhood trauma, depression or repressed desires, problems of the youth and economic insecurity, political instability during adulthood and dieases of old age, etc.

(viii) H. Sequeira (1995) observes the following:

- Yoga teaches one to become passive and tranquil.
- The non-materialistic philosophy of yoga helps one to distinguish between the transitory material situations and the more permanent spiritual dimension of life.
- One has to explore alternative style of living with daily routine of practices, correct diet, a relaxed way of life, capacity to reflect and avoid tense situations and personal philosophy of life for a stress free living.

(ix) B.N. Agarwal (1996) while participating in workshop on "Everybody needs freedom from stress", observed the following:

- Each step in Eight Fold Path (Ashtanga Yoga) of Patanjali aimed at one pointedness and harmonization of the body, mind and spirit.
- Good health is the by-product of yoga and the treatment of disease is not the aim of it. Of course, with the practice of yoga many of the diseases are cured.
- A balanced state of mind is the key to good health and that is possible by integrating certain basic values and concepts in one's life.
- Ahara (diet), Acara (habits), Vihara (recreation) and Vicara (thinking patterns) have to be of a correct type if good health is to be maintained. Yoga and religion lay stress on these aspects of life for attaining good health.

(x) Dr. Sadanand Hulsure (1995) a General Surgeon who himself was once a patient of hyperacidity, chronic cough the inguinal hernia, cured himself through yogic practices in dietary habits, routines, thinking patterns and attitudes. He accepts that his new found insights in yoga had revolutionized his life.

(xi) Dr. S. Shelty (1995) says that the idea of "Dharma" retaining a sense of duty to oneself and being able to be at peace at all times could be achieved. Further he says that devoting a few minutes for oneself, quietening oneself and doing the Asanas (yogic exercises) with correct attitude can be of great help to maintain good health.

3.3 Therapeutic Practices for Relieving Tension

After having a brief survey of research studies, some therapeutic practices are discussed for one's study and practice. There is common principle in all the religions, mysticism and yogic sciences that spirit/soul is the essence of man. Spirit controls the mind and mind controls they body. All these should work in unison in order to keep good health. Spirituality is all powerful dimension in man's life. Therefore, all the therapeutic practices listed here are based on moral and spiritual dimension of life.

They are subtle, potent and powerful from healing point of view. Some of them are common and overlapping in different religions, faiths, mysticism and yogic sciences, since basic assumptions are the same.

Therapeutic practices can be looked from three stand points:

(i) Cognitive (related to knowledge/wisdom)
(ii) Affective (related to emotions/feeling)
(iii) Cognitive/psychomotor (related to action/work)

Accordingly, three broad yogic systems suiting to one's temperament can be practised for drawing the benefit. They are as under:

(i) Jnana yoga (path of wisdom)
(ii) Bhakti yoga (path of devotion)
(iii) Karma yoga (path of action)

In addition to the three listed above, Raja yoga (path of contemplation) without accepting any pre-notion of belief or dogma can also be adopted for attaining higher level of consciousness. As a result, it leads to healing or cure since concentration and control of mind is the central factor here.

Following therapeutic practices can be useful for reducing mental tension.

(i) Naam Japa: Man's word is spirit in man. Spoken words are sounds occasioned by vibrations of thoughts. The "Word" is life energy or cosmic vibratory force. The "mouth of God" is the medulla oblongata in the posterior part of brain, tapering off into the spinal cord. This, the most vital part of the human body is the divine entrance (mouth of God) for the word or life energy, by which man is sustained. In Sikhism, Sri Guru Nanak has shown a path of "Naam Japa". Man can realise God through recitation of divine word. (Sabda Cosmic sound). By communion with Sabda, one can attain the status of siddha (a man of supernatural powers), a Pir (a Muslim divine), a Sura (God) or a Nath (an adept in Yoga). In Hindu, Sikh, Christian and Islamic scriptures the sabda (word) possesses potent power that heals man spiritually. Naam Japa or Mantra Japa (recitation of concentrated divine words) has been accepted as a spiritual therapy in different religions/ faiths and yogic systems.

(ii) Faith: The dictionary meaning of the word "faith" is confidence or trust. Here faith is refered to "higher reality" or "supreme soul" or "greater power" or God. The only method to increase our faith is constantly recalling God whether it be at good or bad times. Even in bad times, we recall God with deep faith in Him. There is an instant feeling of betterment. Absolute, unquestioning faith in God is the greatest method of instantaneous healing. An unceasing effort to arouse that faith is man's highest and most rewarding duty. Reading scriptures or good books and keeping good company (satsang) help to develop/deepen faith and thus elevate level of spiritual energy. Always having a feeling that all that happens is for our good and God is always beside us has a therapeutic value. Faith is the sublime quality that can bring peace in one's life. Lord Sri Krishna has said in the Gita that whoever remembers me at the time of death attains my nature. This illustrates the dictum, you think about God, you become Godly.

(iii) Surrender to the will of God: Psychologically surrendering to the will of God is a very important principle for man. When one surrenders to anyone whether it is a Guru or God or supreme power, the tension becomes less automatically. Therefore, humility and ego surrendering is recommended for removing tension.

(iv) Meditation: Alongwith psychoanalysis and psychiatry, meditation offers solutions to health problems. When one meditates, the doors of one's unconscious level of mind are opened. In the process, one unfolds one's fantasies which play for a while and then disappear. Without knowing, while being in the state of meditation, one has corrected oneself. The individual has overcome his illness and has changed his behaviour.

Meditation is the state where one looks at himself, and into himself and without knowing it, he is cured. According to Eric Fromm what the majority of psychological patients really need is a reorientation of their human destiny so as to become aware of the meaning of life. This is what meditation offers.

(v) Pranayama: Pranayama is a process of control and regulation of breath. There are various techniques and methods in pranayama starting with simple breathing to complex processes of control on breath.

Through pranayama, the process of oxygenation is activated and nerve centres including brain cells get proper blood supply. Not only blood is purified but also thought is harmonised with breath. It helps to release tension.

(vi) Recreation: Recreation is an effective technique to create energy and remove tension. Modes of recreation can be adopted to one's age, liking and temperament. Play, sharing, reading, discussion, painting, listening divine music are some of the ways for man's recreation. Cathersis and expression of emotions help in releasing tension.

(vii) Sleeps, Rest & Relaxation: Human activity leads to stress and tension. On the other hand sleep, rest and relaxation reduce stress and tension. Sleep and rest are the biological needs. Whereas relaxation is a deliberate attempt to reduce tension. Meditative postures and relaxation asanas like shavasana, makarasana and nispandbhava are quite useful for releasing tension. 15 minutes relaxation through shavasana recoups enough energy for the 5/6 hours work. Besides, it has a therapeutic value for the person who practices it.

(viii) Yogic Asanans & Kiryas: Practice of yogic asanas regulates energy in the nerves and glandular systems. Whereas kiryas remove toxins from the body and thus sharpens the functioning of sense organs. Both the practices help in releasing stress and tension from body-mind complex.

(ix) Work: Virtuous action rendered for the welfare of humanity is an effective medium of relaxation and happiness. Day to day work rendered or completed as a duty with commitment and sincerity helps to create an atmosphere of goodwill and welfare. Besides it leads to self-fulfilment and self-actualisation. An attitude of Nishkama Karma (doing action without looking for the fruit) has therapeutic effect on man.

(x) Positive Attitude: Many times stress is caused by our negative attitude towards life. Negative emotions like jealousy, anxiety, fear, anger, attachment create toxins in the body whereas positive bhavas (feelings and emotions) like love, contentment, compassion, sympathy, fellow-feeling, secrete harmones which help to maintain positive health. Positive attitude towards work, people, society and self has a therapeutic effect on man.

Concluding it can be said that holistic approach towards life and living with deep faith in self and God is the safest way to lead tension free life.

References

1. Khosla, D.N. (1988). The Sikh Gurus on Education, Adi-Jugadi Prakashan, Delhi.
2. Jaggi, O.P. (1984). Mental Tension and Its Cure, Orient Paperbacks, Delhi.
3. Swami Tapasyananda, (1987). The Four Yogas of Swami Vivekananda, Advaita Ashrama, 5 Delhi Entally Road, Calcutta.
4. Elenjimittam (1974). The Yoga Philosophy of Patanjali, Hetter Yourself Books, Allahabad.
5. Patel Grish, Heart Disease and Meditation, Prajapita Brahma Kumaris Vishwa–Vidyalaya, New Delhi.
6. -do- (1994) Holistic Health Care, -do-
7. Sinha Phulgenda, (1977). Yoga for Mental Power, Orient Puperbacks, Delhi.
8. Swami Satprakashananda (1976). Meditation: Its Process, Practice, and Culmination, Sri Ramakrishna Math Mylapore, Madras.
9. Yoga and Total Health, Vol. XXXI No. 8, March, 1986 Yoga Institute, Bombay.
10. -do-, Vol. No. XXX, No. 1, 1984.
11. -do-, Vol. No. XXXIII, No. 2, Sept. 1987.
12. -do-, Vol. XXXVI, No. 5, Dec. 1990.
13. -do-, Vol. XXXVIII, No. 6, Jan. 1993.
14. -do-, Vol. XL, No. 2, Sept. 1994.
15. -do-, Vol. XL, No. 2, Oct. 1994.
16. -do-, Vol. XL, No. 12, July, 1995.
17. -do-, Vol. XL1, No. 1, August, 1995.

"क्रोध दुःख की खान है, योग निदान"

चन्द्र भूषण सिंह

क्रोध दुःख के चेतन कारण से उत्पन्न होता है। यह शान्ति भंग करने वाला मनोविकार है। एक क़ा क्रोध दूसरे में भी क्रोध का संचार करता है। जिसके प्रति क्रोध–प्रदर्शन होता है वह तत्काल अपमान का अनुभव करता है और इस दुःख पर उसकी भो त्यौरी चढ़ जाती है। यह विचार करने वाले बहुत थोड़े निकलते हैं कि हम पर जो क्रोध प्रकट किया जा रहा है, वह उचित है या अनुचित। इसी से धर्म, नीति और शिष्टाचार तीनों में क्रोध के निरोध का उपदेश पाया जाता है। संत लोग जो खलों में क्रोध के वचन सहते ही हैं, गृहस्थ लोग भी न जाने कितनी ऊँची–नीची पचाते रहते हैं। सभ्यता के व्यवहार में भी क्रोध नहीं तो क्रोध के चिन्ह दबाये जाते हैं। इस प्रकार का प्रतिबन्ध समाज के सुख–शान्ति के लिए बहुत आवश्यक है।

क्रोध मन को एक उत्तेजित और खिंची हुई स्थिति में रख देता है जिसके परिणामस्वरूप मन दुषित विकारों से भर जाता है। क्रोध से प्रथम तो उद्वेग उत्पन्न होता है। रक्त में गरमी आ जाती है और उसका प्रवाह बड़ा तेज हो जाता है। इस गरमी से मनुष्य के शुभ–भाव–प्रेम, सत्य, न्याय, विवेक, बुद्धि आदि जल जाते हैं।

क्रोध एक प्रकार का भूत है, जिसके सवार होते ही मनुष्य अपने में नहीं रहता। उस पर किसी दूसरी सत्ता का प्रभाव हो जाता है। मन की निन्द्य वृत्तियाँ उस पर अपनी राक्षसी माया चढ़ा देती है, वह बेचारा इतना हतबुद्धि हो जाता है कि उसे यह ज्ञान ही नहीं रहता कि वह क्या कर रहा है।

क्रोध का वेग इतना प्रबल होता है कि कभी–कभी मनुष्य यह भी विचार नहीं करता कि जिसने दु:ख पहुँचाया है, उसमें दु:ख पहुँचाने की इच्छा भी थी या नहीं। इसी से कभी तो वह अचानक पैर कुचल जाने पर किसी को मार बैठता है और कभी ठोकर खाकर कंकड़–पत्थर तोड़ने लगता है। चाणक्य ब्राह्मण अपना विवाह करने जाता था। मार्ग में कुश उसके पैर में चुभे। वह चट मट्ठा और कुदाली लेकर पहुँचा और कुशों को उखाड़ कर उनकी जड़ों में मट्ठा देने लगा। एक बार एक ब्राह्मण देवता चूल्हा फूँकते–फूँकते थक गये। जब आग न जली तब उस पर क्रोध करके चूल्हे में पानी डाल किनारे हो गये इस प्रकार का क्रोध अपरिस्कृत है। यात्रियों ने ऐसे बहुत से जंगलियों का हाल लिखा है जो रास्ते में पत्थर की ठोकर लगने पर बिना उसको चूर–चूर किये आगे नहीं बढ़ते। अधिक अभ्यास के कारण यदि कोई मनोविकार बहुत प्रबल पड़ जाता है, तो वह अन्त: प्रकृति में अव्यवस्था उत्पन्न कर मनुष्य को बचपन से मिलती–जुलती अवस्था में ले जाकर पटक देता है।

क्रोध सब मनोविकारों से फुर्तिला है, इसी से अवसर पड़ने पर वह और मनोविकारों का भी साथ देकर उनकी तुष्टि का साधक होता है। कभी वह दया के साथ कूदता है, कभी घृणा के। एक क्रूर कुमार्गी किसी अनाथ अबला पर अत्याचार कर रहा है। हमारे हृदय में उस अनाथ अबला के प्रति दया उमड़ रही है। पर दया की अपनी शक्ति तो त्याग और कोमल व्यवहार तक होती है। यदि वह स्त्री अर्थकष्ट में होती तो उसे कुछ देकर हम अपनी दया के वेग को देकर शान्त कर लेते। पर यहाँ तो उस अबला के दु:ख का कारण मूर्तिमान तथा अपनी विरूद्ध प्रयत्नों को ज्ञानपूर्वक रोकने की शक्ति रखने वाला है। ऐसी अवस्था में क्रोध ही उस अत्याचारी के दमन के लिए उत्तेजित करता है जिसके बिना हमारी दया ही व्यर्थ जाती। क्रोध अपनी इस सहायता के बदले में दया की वाह वाही को नहीं बाँटता। काम क्रोध करता है, पर नाम दया ही का होता है। लोग यही कहते हैं कि ''उसने दया करके बचा लिया'' यह कोई नहीं कहता कि ''क्रोध करके बचा लिया'' ऐसे अवसरों पर यदि क्रोध दया का साथ न दे तो दया अपनी प्रवत्ति के अनुसार परिणाम उपस्थित ही नहीं करती।

यह क्रोध करुणा के आज्ञाकारी सेवक के रूप में हमारे सामने आता है। क्रौंच के वध पर बाल्मिकि मुनि से करुण क्रोध का सौन्दर्य एक महाकाव्य का सौन्दर्य हुआ। उक्त सौन्दर्य का कारण है निर्विशेषता। बाल्मिकि के क्रोध के भीतर प्राणिमात्र के दु:ख की सहानुभूति छिपी है–राम के क्रोध के भीतर सम्पूर्ण लोक के दु:ख का क्षोम समाया हुआ है। क्षमा जहाँ से श्रीहत हो जाती है, वहीं से

क्रोध के सौन्दर्य का आरम्भ होता है। शिशुपाल की बहुत-सी बुराइयों तक जब श्रीकृष्ण की क्षमा पहुँच चुकी तब जाकर सभी-चीनता का सूत्रपात हुआ। अपने ही दुःख पर उत्पन्न क्रोध में या तो हमें तत्काल क्षमा का अवसर या अधिकार ही नहीं रहता अथवा वह अपना प्रभाव खो चुकी रहती है। इस प्रकार का क्रोध वास्तविक योग साधकों का क्रोध हो सकता है वरना मानवी जीवन में क्रोध प्राण हरण करने वाला शत्रु है। आमतौर पर क्रोध को पाप का बाप ही कहा जायेगा।

क्रोधः प्राणहरः शत्रुः क्रोधो मित्रमुखो रिपुः।
क्रोधोह्यसिर्महातीक्ष्णः सर्व क्रोधोडपकर्षति।।
तपते यजते चैव यच्च दानं प्रयच्छाति।
क्रोधेन सर्व हरति तस्मात् क्रोधं विसर्जयेत्।।

(बाल्मिकि रामायण, उत्तर)

अर्थात् 'क्रोध प्राण हरण करने वाला शत्रु है, क्रोध मुंह पर मीठा बोलने वाला बैरी है, क्रोध तप, यज्ञ और दान सभी का हरण कर लेता है। अतएव क्रोध को छोड़ देना चाहिए।

क्रोध का मन के अनन्य विकारों से घनिष्ट सम्बन्ध है। क्रोध के वशीभूत होकर हमें उचित अनुचित का विवेक नहीं रहता और हम हाथा-पाई कर बैठते हैं। बातों-बातों में ही उखड़ जाना लड़ाई करना साधारण-सी बात है यदि तुरन्त क्रोध का निवारण हो जाए, तब तो मानसिक स्वास्थ्य की दृष्टि से ठीक है, पर यदि वह अन्तः प्रदेश में पहुँचकर भावना-ग्रन्थि बन जाय तब तो बड़ा ही दुःखदायी होता है। बहुत दिनों तक टिका हुआ क्रोध वैर कहलाता है। *वैर क्रोध का अचार या मुरब्बा है*। वैर एक ऐसी मानसिक बीमारी है जिसका कुफल मनुष्य को दैनिक जीवन में भुगतना पड़ता है। वह अपने को किसी भी सूरत में संतुलित नहीं रख पाता। जिससे उसका बैर है, उसके उत्तम गुण, भलाई, पुराना प्रेम, उच्च संस्कार इत्यादि सब वह विस्तृत कर बैठता है। स्थायी रूप से एक भावना ग्रन्थि बन जाने से क्रोध का वेग तो धीमा पड़ जाता है, किन्तु दूसरे व्यक्ति को सजा देने नुकसान पहुँचाने या पीड़ित करने की कुक्सित भावना निरन्तर मन को दग्ध किया करती है।

वैर पुरानी जीर्ण मानसिक बीमारी है। क्रोध तत्कालीन और क्षणिक प्रमाद है। क्रोध में पागल होकर मनुष्य सोचने का समय नहीं देखता।

वैर उसके लिए बहुत समय लेता है। क्रोध में अस्थिरता, क्षणिकता, तत्कालीनता, बुद्धि का कुण्ठित हो जाना, उद्विग्नता, आत्मरक्षा, अहंकार की पुष्टि,

असहिष्णुता, दूसरे को दण्डित करने की भावानाएँ संयुक्त हैं। वैर में सोचने-समझने, प्रतिशोध लेने का समय होता है। हम अच्छी तरह सोचते हैं कुछ समय लेते हैं और तब बदला लेते हैं।

पूर्ण क्रोध की अवस्था में मनुष्य दुःख पहुँचाने वाले पात्र की ओर ही उन्मुख रहता है। उसी को भयभीत या पीड़ित करने की चेष्टा में प्रवृत्त रहता है। आवेग में दुःख पहुँचाने वाली बात के ब्यौरों पर और उसकी असह्यता पर विशेष ध्यान रहता है। इसकी ठीक व्यंजना ऐसे वाक्यों में समझनी चाहिए- "तुमने मेरे साथ यह किया, वह किया। तब तक तो मैं सहता आया, अब नहीं सह सकता"। इसके आगे बढ़कर जब कोई धूल में मिला दूँगा, दाँत पीसता और गरजता हुआ यह कहने लगे कि "मैं तुम्हें धूल में मिला दूँगा, तुम्हारा घर खोदकर फेंक दूँगा"। तब क्रोध का पूर्ण स्वरूप समझना चाहिए।

गाँधी जी कहा करते थे कि क्रोध के लक्षण शराब और अफीम दोनों से मिलते हैं। शराबी की भाँति क्रोधी मनुष्य भी पहले लाल पीला होता है, फिर आवेश के मन्द होने पर भी क्रोध न घटा तो वह अफीम का काम करता है और मनुष्य की बुद्धि कुरेद डालता है। क्रोध से क्रमशः सम्मोह, स्मृति भ्रंश और बुद्धिनाश माने गये हैं।

अब प्रश्न यह उठता है कि आखिरकार ऐसी जघन्य बीमारी से कैसे बचा जाये? मनुष्य जब क्रोध के पूर्ण आवेग में होता है तब उसके शरीर व मन की दशा कैसी होती है तथा इस निकृष्ट अवस्था का सूत्रपात कैसे होता है इस पहलुओं पर विचार कर लेना जरूरी है तभी योग विद्या में इसका निदान ढूँढ सकते हैं।

क्रोध उभाड़ की प्रक्रिया

क्रोध उत्पन्न हो गया यह एक मनुष्य की अवस्था है, परन्तु क्रोध को इस अवस्था तक आने में निम्न प्रक्रिया से गुजरना पड़ता है। (कृपया चार्ट देखें)

क्रोध का प्रभाव क्षेत्र

1. **भोजनः** भोजन कितना भी सुस्वायु, पौष्टिक और सुपाच्य हो, परन्तु भोजन के समय खाने वाला ईर्ष्या, क्रोधादि विकारों से ग्रस्त है तो वह उत्तम भोजन भी व्यर्थ जायेगा और शरीर को नहीं लगेगा। मनुस्मृति में कहा गया है:

   पूजयेदशर्ननित्यमद्याच्चैमनकुत्सयन्।
   दृष्ट्वा द्रष्योत्प्रसीदेच्च प्रतिनन्देच्य सर्वशः।।

क्रोध उमाड़ की प्रक्रिया : क्रोध उत्पन्न हो गया। यह एक मनुष्य की अवस्था है, परन्तु क्रोध की इस अवस्था तक आने में निम्न प्रक्रिया से गुजरना पड़ता है।

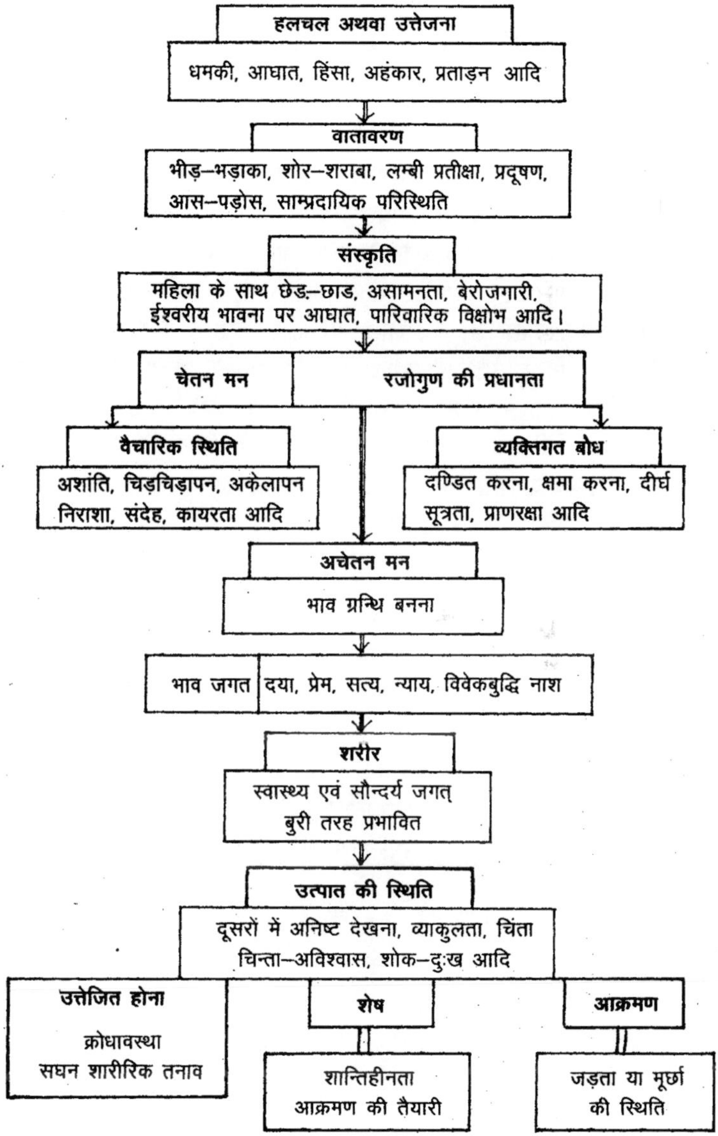

अर्थात् भोजन का पूजन करके खाना चाहिए। भगवान के पूजन में जैसी पवित्रता और स्वच्छता का ध्यान रखा जाता है, वैसा ही भोजन के प्रति रखना चाहिए। विज्ञान ने भी सिद्ध किया है कि क्रोध एवं व्याकुल चित्त से खाया गया पौष्टिक भोजन भी हानि करता है। इसलिए भोजन के समय क्रोध, भय, विषाद, घृणा आदि विकार मन में नहीं रखना चाहिए। जो कुछ भी सामने आवे उसको भगवान का प्रसाद मानकर खाना चाहिए और कभी भी भोजन की निन्दा नहीं करनी चाहिए।

2. **शरीर की स्थितिः** क्रोध उत्पन्न होने पर शरीर में अभूतपूर्व आकस्मिक परिवर्तन होता है। क्रोधी व्यक्ति का मुखमण्डल कैसा हो जाता है, जरा शीशे में देखे तो पता चलता है। कैसा मुख लाल हो जाता है, कटुशब्दों का उच्चारण करने से शरीर काँपने लगता है, भुजाएँ फड़कने लगती हैं। भृकुटी चढ़ जाती है, नेत्र लाल हो जाते हैं, होंठ चलने लगते हैं। मन में उद्वेग, विकलता, गवै उग्रता इत्यादि अनुभव उदय होते हैं। प्रत्येक मानसिक व्यापार या क्रिया का सम्बन्ध चेहरे के सौन्दर्य से है। मन के विकार का प्रभाव शरीर के अवयवों पर लक्षित होता है। प्राण शक्ति का क्षय होता है, शरीर-यन्त्र गतिहीन हो जाता है, मनुष्य पशु तुल्य बन जाता है तथा शरीर का सौन्दर्य ही नष्ट हो जाता है।

3. **स्वास्थ्यः** क्रोधी मनुष्य कभी स्वस्थ नहीं रह सकता। उसका चेहरा पीला पड़ जाता है। शरीर सूख कर कांटा हो जाता है। पाचन-शक्ति तो बिल्कुल ही बिगड़ जाती है जिसके फलस्वरूप शरीर रोगों का घर बन जाता है। क्रोधी मनुष्य की नाड़ी की गति तेज हो जाती है। नशें ऊपर की ओर खड़ी हुई दिखाई देती हैं। क्रोधावेश में वह दाँत पीसने लगता है उसकी साँस जल्दी-जल्दी चलने लगती है, भौहें और हाथ सिकुड़ने लगते हैं। उसका शरीर रोमांचित हो जाता है, जबान खुश्क हो जाती है और खून में गरमी पैदा हो जाती है। एड्रिनल ग्रन्थि से अत्याधिक एड्रेनलिन का स्राव होने लगता है जो खून में मिलकर जिगर में पहुँचता है जिससे शरीर के अंगों में बेचैनी उत्पन्न होती है। साथ ही रग और पुट्ठों में बहुत खिंचावट पैदा करती है। ईर्ष्या और क्रोध दोनों दाहक हैं। देह और मन को जलाते हैं। मनुष्य को पनपने का अवसर नहीं देते। क्रोध से बनी विचार-मूर्तियाँ नीचे ऊपर, मानस-पटल के प्रत्येक कोने पर छा जाती हैं और उसे मोहाच्छन्न कर देती हैं। इन विचार-मूर्तियों में एक प्रकार का कम्पन होता रहता है तथा ये जैसी हैं वैसी ही किरणें निकलती रहती हैं। साथ ही जैसे ये

विचार–मूर्तियाँ हमाने मानसिक जगत में बनी हैं, वैसी ही, उसी क्षण जिसके निमित्त ये बनी हैं, उसकी ओर दौड़ जाती हैं।

4. **संस्कारः** क्रोध मनुष्य जीवन का निकृष्ट कर्म है। इसका कुफल हमारे जीवन को प्रभावित करता है। हम जो कर्म करते हैं उसका परिणाम तो भुगतना ही है, चाहे वर्तमान में भुगतें अथवा भविष्य में। हमारे कर्मों का प्रभाव ही संस्कारों को जन्म देता है। हमारे अन्दर पूर्व जन्म के संस्कार भी होते हैं और वर्तमान भी हम कर्मो के आचरण से नये संस्कार धारण करते हैं। ईर्ष्या, क्रोध प्रमाद उद्वेग, विकलता आदि मनोविकार हमारे कर्मों में भोजन के नमक की तरह घुल कर रक्त में घूमते रहते हैं और अवसर आने पर वे सम्पूर्ण शरीर को अपने प्रभाव क्षेत्र में ले लेते हैं। जिससे हमारे अच्छे संस्कार दब जाते हैं और क्रोधाग्नि की आँच से झुलस जाते हैं। फलस्वरूप हम मन का शील, मधुरता, सौन्दर्य की अनुभूति उत्तम स्वभाव, शुभ भावनाएँ तथा आध्यात्मिक सजीवनता से पूर्ण वंचित रह जाते हैं।

क्रोध का यौगिक निदान

षड् दोषाः पुरूषेणेह हातव्या भूतिमिच्छता।
निद्रा तन्द्रा भयं क्रोध आलस्यं दीर्घसूलता।।

अर्थात् निद्रा, तन्द्रा, भय, क्रोध, आलस्य और दीर्घसूत्रता–ये चरित्र के छः दोष मनुष्य की उन्नति के बाधक हैं। अतः उन्नति चाहने वाले पुरूष को इनका सर्वथा त्याग कर देना चाहिए।

अंधा वह नहीं, जिसकी आँखे फूट गयी हैं। अंधा वह है, जो क्रोधी है। क्रोध के आवेग को रोकने के लिए स्वास्थ्यमय शुभेच्छाओं एवं मधुरता से अपने मन को सजाना चाहिए। अपनी शक्तियों में श्रद्धा, पापों से सावधानी, प्रभु पर विश्वास वे गुण हैं। इनसे क्रोध का उफान कम होता है तथा चित्त शान्त होता है।

क्रोध से बचने का स्थायी और वास्तविक उपाय योग साधना में निहित है। निरन्तर योग साधना करने वाले व्यक्ति का मन स्थिर और शान्त हो जाता है। संसार की घटनाएँ उसे विचलित नहीं कर पातीं। वह अपने इर्द–गिर्द होने वाली घटनाओं को साक्षी भाव से देखने में समर्थ हो जाता है। वह क्रोध में भी अवस्था का साक्षी बन जाता है। वह ऐसे दुःखों से घबराता नहीं है। उसके विचार और व्यवहार संतुलित और समरस हो जाते हैं। उसकी वाणी में मधुरता आ जाती

है। योग-ध्यान आदि के अभ्यास से हमारे शरीर की पूरी रासायनिक रचना में परिवर्तन आ जाता है। इन परिवर्तनों के कारण ईर्ष्या, क्रोध, भय, आलस्य आदि मनोविकार नष्ट हो जाते हैं तथा शारीरिक मानसिक स्वास्थ्य की पूर्णता आने लगती है। बेचैन मनुष्य मानसिक द्वन्द्व, संघर्ष और तनाव से मुक्त हो जाता है।

समस्त शारीरिक-मानसिक विकारों को दूर करने के लिए हठयोग, जप, त्राटक, ध्यान, निष्पन्दभाव, सात्विक आहार, यम-नियम आदि का मार्ग ही श्रेष्ठ साधन है।

तत्काल क्रोध पर नियन्त्रण कैसे?

जैसे ही क्रोध उत्पन्न हो तो व्यक्ति को निम्न उपाय करना चाहिए:

1. क्रोध आने पर मौन रहना उचित है। जिसके प्रति क्रोध आया है, उसके समीप न रहिए।
2. क्रोध के लक्षण दीखने पर घने वृक्ष के नीचे अलग जा बैठिये।
3. क्रोध उत्पन्न होते ही शीतल जल पीना चाहिए तथा मुँह पर पानी के छीटें देकर धो लेना चाहिए।
4. लम्बा गहरा शीतली क्रिया करें तथा अपने श्वास का निरीक्षण करें।
5. कोई प्रिय भजन, कीर्तन अथवा नाम सुमिरन करें।
6. किसी इष्ट मित्र के साथ घुल मिलकर बातें करें।
7. सुन्दर मनोवैज्ञानिक लेख पढ़ें जिससे शान्ति प्राप्त हो।
8. दर्पण के सामने खड़े होकर अपने मुख मण्डल को देखें।

मेरा मुझमें कुछ नहीं, जो कछु है सो तेरा।
तेरा तुझको सौंप दूं, क्या लागे है मेरा।।

इसी समर्पित भाव के साथ स्वयं को समर्पित करता हूँ। क्रोध से मुक्ति पाइये। पहले जरा आप मुस्कुराइये।

Part III

YOGA, EDUCATION, PHYSICAL EDUCATION AND SPORTS

Redefining Yogic Education

Swami Niranjanananda Saraswati

We have had to re-think and re-define the goals of people involved in and trying to propagate yoga. In the time of our guru, Paramahamsa Satyananda, the propagation of yoga took the form of introducing yoga to a broad range of people in different countries and cultures. He started off a trend which took us beyond the superficial dimension into a deeper understanding of what yoga has to offer and how it could be applied in our lives. In 1983 I was put in a tight spot; I went from being a free, independent swami to looking after the entire organization. It took me eleven years to know how to carry on the work of yoga.

When certain ideas became clear, we started a new approach to yogic education with the formation of a Yoga University, the first one of its kind in the world. The seed of this undertaking was planted in November 1993 during the World Yoga Convention, which was organized in Munger to commemorate the fifty years of renunciation and service to humanity of Paramahamsa Satyananda. The university will provide ample scope for studying, understanding and applying the subtle aspects of yoga.

The concept of yoga has changed with the times. In Britain, during the early sixties, there was a yoga teacher by the name of Richard Hittleman who taught yoga on TV for beautifying the body. At that time, in Australia, Roma Blair was teaching yoga for physical fitness and reduction of the waistline. Swami Sarasvati, who is not related to us, also came up with her brand cf yoga in Australia. That period of yogic propagation was confined to the aspect of asana for the physical body, because the whole concept was new. Nobody taught pranayama or even knew what it was. Pranayama was considered to the type of breathing exercise that is very difficult and dangerous to do. Nobody had ever heard of mudra, bandha or shatkarma, of kriya yoga, raja yoga, bhakti yoga or karma yoga for that matter.

Later on the concept and the thrust of yoga changed. It became a way to attain mental relaxation, to reduce stress and anxiety, to find some form of mental peace, with the emergence of Transcendental Meditation (TM). Then many different groups and individuals adopted the yogic structure and created their own brand of yoga. In the present day, a new approach to yoga is emerging. Yoga has not changed. The practices, theories and concepts are the same, but our acceptance, understanding and application are changing. In the modern context, the need to look deeper into yoga has become more evident. As we find ourselves thrown into conflict in relation to our society, family and work, we lose our balance, inner peace and harmony. Despite these influences, which are both external and internal, we are looking into a method whereby we can integrate our personality. This integration is the main thrust of yoga teaching.

Law of Karma

Today society is at a crossroads and such institutions as the Yoga University are necessary so that we can learn to deal with life in a more positive, systematic and balanced way. Until now, due to lack of understanding and awareness, we have been misusing the potential and the faculties of our life. In order to overcome the feeling of guilt, we say that life is all a play of karma, that it is our karma to be like this or like that. However, the law of totally different to our limited concept, no matter what people may say about it.

Karma represented the continuity of action which is performed by an individual on the physical, mental and emotional levels. Our thoughts are karmas; they are actions of the mind. Feelings are karmas of the heart. Ambitions are karmas of the ego. Wherever there is some form of manifestation, an idea taking a form even if it is within our mind, it is a karma. The *Bhagavad Gita* has stated that each individual performs karmas not only through the body and the senses, but also through the mind, emotions, interactions and beliefs. However, there also has to be a process of elimination and we do not know this technique.

How can we eliminate the negative karmas? Let me give you an example. We eat, we digest the food and afterwards, what do we do? Bring it out the other way. There is a process of natural elimination; it is a law. Whatever you eat and drink has to come out, you cannot hold it inside. If You try, you will become badly constipated. This law also applies to our mental body. We are constantly feeding ourselves through our emotions, through a search for fulfilment, pleasure, satisfaction and contentment. However, we are not able to eliminate what has already been digested, and what is not eliminated is accumulated inside. This accumulation of mental toxins has to be eliminated and the elimination is known as purification of inner karma.

Trend of Modern Therapies

We contain both positive and negative qualities. Negative qualities are the tamasic, restrictive, detrimental qualities, which inhibit the growth and flowering of life. The positive qualities are rajasic and aid the process of growth in life. In the absence of such recognition, our inner body which is comprised of mind *(manas)*, intellect *(buddhi)*, memory *(chitta)* and ego *(ahamkara)*, is in a state of imbalance. This state of imbalance creates physical, emotional and mental disturbance which later manifests in the form of disease and illness.

Modern therapies are trying desperately to find a way to promote health, but their concept of health promotion is very superficial. They look at the body, at the disease which has already taken hold and try to rectify that. I remember a story about a great statesman. He was eleven and lived with his mother on a farm. There were many plants, trees and shrubs which were cared for by his mother. Once she had to leave the farm for several days and so she asked her son to look after the plants while she was away. The son said, 'Fine, it is a very simple job. I can do it.'

When the mother returned she saw that all her plants were wilted; the flowers had fallen off and the leaves were drooping. Seeing their conditions, she called for son and asked him, 'How did you look after the plants?' He replied, 'Everyday I went around with a cloth and cleaned each plant very carefully, every leaf, every flower petal, the trunk or stem. I made sure there was not a single speck of dust and if I found any insects, I killed them. Every morning I polished the fruit on the tree.' The mother asked one question. 'Did you ever water the plants?' The son said, 'No, I forgot!'

This is also the story of our lives. When we get a pimple or a mosquito bite, we apply a spray. We look after the tree externally, but we are not able to provide water for the roots which are unseen. This has been the trend of modern therapies. They look at that portion of the tree which is above the ground. If the tree is sick, if bugs are eating the leaves, they spray it and kill and the bugs. That is the most crude form of treatment. Many people are now going back to an organic life-style, but still our vision has not changed. Maybe the methods of treating our problems have changed, but the approach has not.

Samskara

Yoga says, 'Don't observe only the trunk, branches, leaves and fruits'. Of course, they are there and we have to look after them, but they are not the main point of focus. We also have to care for the roots which are underground. If we cannot provide the roots with water, sooner or later the tree is going to die. This is what happens in the course of life. We live life, but we are dead people. We are not alive, vibrant, expressing our creativity and joy. We are caught up in the negative emotions which have accumulated in our heads and which have full control over our actions, behaviour and thinking. These negative emotions or karmas, actions which have left their imprint in the mind-field, have to be eliminated.

In order to go through this process of elimination, we have to educate ourselves in yoga. The trend in society today is towards job-oriental education. When we go to school, we have to make a projection about what we wish to become in the future. Then we have to learn those skills which will be useful for the future. This is a form of externalized education, but we are missing something vital. Our education has taught us how to look after the trunk, branches, leaves and fruit, but it has not taught us about imbibing samskara.

The word *samskara* has been defined as mental programming or conditioning, according to which we act and live, but that is not the actual meaning. Samskara is derived from two roots; *akara* means a form, a complete image; and *sam* means balanced. So the literal meaning of samskara is a balanced, harmonious, integrated image which we need to develop about ourselves. This image is imbibed through yoga.

Cause of Suffering

When we are unable to eliminate the negative mind stuff, then we suffer and this suffering can take any form. It can take the form of physical disease, mental imbalance, emotional crisis or spiritual crisis due to suppression and misunderstanding in life. Yogis knew that suffering would increase in the future. Yogis are thinkers who are able to apply certain aspects of yoga in order to improve the conditions of normal life. In fact, in the literature of tantra or yoga such as *Gherand Samhita* and *Hatha Yoga Pradipika,* it is clear that there is a dialogue between two people, one asking a question and the other giving the answer. The question is: how to overcome suffering?

Suffering has been divided into three categories: *(i) adidevic, (ii) adibhautic,* and *(iii) adhyatmic.* The first is adidevic which means suffering due to natural causes such as earthquake, flood, famine, fire and other catastrophes over which there is no human control. The second is adibhautic which means suffering which is generated due to wrong life-style, to lack of understanding of how to live in the right way, and to changing situations, in the world which are not able to adjust or cope with. Adibhautic suffering includes most of the diseases and illnesses which we encounter today. The third category is adhyatmic suffering which is due to spiritual causes.

How to overcome suffering

The three kinds of suffering which have been defined in yogic literature are natural, personal and spiritual. The way given to overcome this suffering is through a process of working with the different areas of our personality. In yoga this process is called sadhana. Whatever form of meditation we do, whether it is self-observation, antar mouna, ajapa japa, dharana or yoga nidra, these different yogic sadhanas deal with the human mind. They relate to and harmonize the aspect of chitta.

Karma yoga relates with the actions that we perform in life. When karma yoga becomes natural, spontaneous and effortless, we will develop immunity to action. Karma yoga is not the yoga of action, rather it is a way to develop immunity to the effects and influences of action. If I say something bad, you will not like it. If I say something good, you will like it. That means you are not immune to what I am saying. What I am saying is an action being performed by me, and how you are receiving it is your reaction to my action.

If we are able to develop immunity to the negative influences, the tamasic tendencies of life, then karma becomes karma yoga. Otherwise, it is only a head trip, an intellectual concept that we are doing karma yoga, that karma yoga means hard work or a change of attitude. Karma yoga is not a change of attitude, hard work or selfless service. It is a method by which we can develop immunity in life, and his immunity relates to the aspect of manas which is responsible for interaction, for our external behaviour. We constantly analyze our behaviour, how we are going to perform so that other people will accept us as nice people. That behaviour is related to manas.

Other yogic sadhanas, such as the meditative practices of pratyahara and dharana, influence the aspect of chitta. Jnana yoga is not study, rather it is applying what we know in life. This application influences the aspect of buddhi, and it is not easy. Many times we know that whatever we wish to do is not possible at present. We feel certain conflicts; we wish to lead our life in a certain way but we cannot. We have the knowledge but we are not able to apply it. When we begin to live that understanding, that knowledge, then jnana yoga influences the aspect of buddhi, and buddhi is harmonized. The harmony of manas, buddhi and chitta helps to organize the structure of ahamkara or ego.

Yogic Education

We have to re-define our understanding of yoga and yogic education because we work at many subtle levels. Our roots are what actually support us. If the roots die, the tree is not going to survive. Awareness and harmonization of these roots leads to the elimination of mental toxins. At present we do not have the ability to release what we feel or what we have accumulated mentally because we are not aware of ourselves. I know that I am not aware and if I, who continuously think about yoga and how to present it, am not aware, then how can another person who just comes in contact with yoga for an hour every day be aware?

An adjustment has to take place. It is the acceptance, conditioning and expression of life, and the accommodation of human karmas in life which is the aim of yoga. People talk about very nice concepts and theories of transcendence, no doubt, but we have to begin by providing ourselves with an education which makes us aware of our inner personality. In the first sutra of Patanjali, "*Atha yogaanushasanam*", it states that 'the aim of yoga is to govern the subtle structure of human personality'.

If we can understand this much and expand it in our own way, what will happen? When our subtle, inner personality is harmonized, how will we function? How will we think? How will we behave? How will we act? What will we express? It will be totally different to what we are experiencing right now. It is that self-education where we become aware of ourselves, not a job-oriented education, that yoga propagates. This awareness is incredible. The mind has infinite possibilities and because we are an expression, an extension of that mind in the external world, we have infinite possibilities.

Yogic Psychotherapy

These infinite possibilities are the result of attaining higher consciousness, progressively increasing our state of awareness. It is the increasing states of awareness which change the quality of life. The yogic theories about kundalini yoga represent the changing, evolving quality of life. In its description of the chakras, kundalini yoga has come forward as the most effective psychotherapy ever to exist on this planet. At first we deal with the mooladhara level of consciousness where we take up that aspects of security and insecurity. The idea of security in life is very strong. We do not want to become insecure; we want to maintain our stability. However, in order to maintain stability, we have to latch on to something in the absence of which we again become insecure.

So, the whole aspect of mind and consciousness in relation to security and insecurity becomes a very vicious circle. Again the effect of karma comes in. While travelling from one country to the next, especially in Europe, often I would get funny feelings in my heart because I did not change gear. If people like what I say, they like it; if they do not like it, they do not. I think that if I were to adjust my thinking according to the mentalities of everyone, my life would be a living hell. So I do not adjust with anyone's mentality; I live as I am. But because of this I would often get such thoughts as, 'Will I be admitted into this country or not?'

Once I went to Greece which is a very orthodox country. They do not like any threat to their security and they held me at the airport for six hours because they wanted to deport me. I think the customs officer had got out of the wrong side of the bed because I had given him my most special smile and it had not worked. For the first few moments I realized what anxiety was. The fear of deportation, of not being allowed into the country was very strong although I had done nothing, somebody just did not life my face or dress.

I said to myself, 'What is this? Why am I reacting this way? and I started doing my mantra. There was another lady in a similar situation. She was in her fifties and I was eighteen. While we were waiting for the decision, I sat down very comfortably on the sofa with my mala and started to do japa, passing the time. The lady was pacing up and down, up and down, up and down. I wanted her for some time until I had to close my eyes as they had become like a pendulum. She was smoking continuously and after every packet she would ask me, 'Aren't you nervous?'

I said, 'I was nervous but not anymore. Walking around the room is not going to help me enter the country. Smoking five packets of cigarettes in one hour is not going to help me enter the country. If I have to enter, I will enter, if I don't, I won't. I will still get to sit on the plane and enjoy a good flight.' I think it was a test of God who finally said, 'This fellow has passed the test of mooladhara, insecurity, so let him through.' Then God changed the programming of the customs officer and I was in.

From that day I started to think about the experiences that people have when they encounter insecurities, fears, traumas and distractions in life. Because we encounter many different experiences, we are not able to get a grip on our nature. The yogic concept of kundalini yoga in relation to the chakras deals with this specific subject. Kundalini is not a serpent which rises from mooladhara and goes up to sahasrara. It is a symbol of passing through different states of consciousness, from first into second, into third, into fourth. This process continues all the way through. As we pass each layer of our consciousness, we come to realize how we have been responding to a certain situation and how we can harmonize that.

Mooladhara represents insecurity in the negative aspect and security in the positive aspect. Swadhisthana represents fear in the negative aspect and absence of fear in the positive aspect. Manipura represents the dissipated nature in the negative aspect–too much happening, to much dynamism, uncontrolled activity of the brain and mind, of the emotions and feelings. In the positive aspect manipura represents a state of observation where everything is being performed in the right way. You are in tune with yourself, with your personality, with the environment, with nature and with the divine will.

Anahata in the negative aspect represents distorted or adulterated feelings, in the sense that too many things have left their mark and we are not able to experience the real nature of feeling. In the positive sense anahata represents clean feeling.

Adjustment in Life

In this way we work through each level of consciousness, eliminating the accumulated toxins. Every moment of the day becomes the practice of yoga, not only the hour which we spend in the classroom. If we can observe ourselves and through this process of observation harmonize ourselves, that is the real yoga–observation and harmonization. Then yoga becomes a practice which we perform every moment of the day. It is not something we do at a given time and then forget. That is the real essence of yoga and the theory behind yogic education. Yogic education, which is self-education, has to be combined with the life-styles. We do not have to alter anything externally. It is only question of a positive adjustment in life.

Paramahamsa Satyananda once said, 'We say we suffer, we say we have pain, and we try to find a solution. If we look around we will not find any solution to that suffering or pain. However, the solution comes naturally when we are able to adjust to the suffering and pain. If we can adjust to suffering then it ceases to be suffering. If we can adjust to pain then it ceases to be pain. There is no such thing as pain or pleasure; it is a symptom of adjustment.' If we think critically about this statement of Paramahamsaji's, we will find it to be a very precise, definite and true statement which we can apply in our own life situations. It is this process of adjustment that we learn through yoga.

Two approaches of yoga

So, we have to think about how to incorporate yoga into our life-style. We can start off with our immediate needs. Do we need yoga because we suffer from a physical or a mental problem, because we lack something in our life? Whatever the reason, that should become a stepping stone for us to actually experience yoga in our lives. We can use yoga in the case of illness. However, we should remember that the doctor gives medicine while the patient is ill and the medicine has to be taken until the patient reaches good health. After taking the medicine and becoming well, there is no need to continue with it. The same principle applies in yoga. We do not have to practise the complete system of yoga everyday. We do not have to practice asana and pranayama; they are practised in order to rectify certain imbalances. We can forget about these practices unless we require them and just live yoga from moment to moment.

These are the two approaches of yoga. One incorporates physical involvement, every morning practising asana, pranayama, relaxation, meditation and mantra. Then the rest of the day one can practise the yoga of awareness in order to eliminate the accumulated mental toxins. This is how yoga has to be done. So, we have two commitments to ourselves. The first is to become physically well, for which SYTREC and different ashrams are available. The second aspect is to become internally well. This education which teaches us about becoming internally well can be acquired in an ashram environment where one is exposed to a yogic life-style. We have to expose ourselves to a yogic life-style and see how this applies in our present condition. Only then can yoga become a part of us. This is what we hope to achieve in a more professional and determined way with the establishment of the Yoga University.

Education should prepare us for an ideal life.
Smile with the flowers and green grass.
Play with the birds and the deer.
Shake hands with the ferns and twigs.
Talk to the rainbow, wind, stars and the sun.
Converse with the running brook and the waves of the sea.
Develop friendship with all your neighbours, dogs, cats, trees and flowers.
Then You will have a wide, perfect and full life.

—Swami Sivananda

Evaluation of Yoga Education

S.P. Duggal

1. Bases of Evaluation : Objectives

For proper evaluation, it is imperative to clearly perceive the purpose of carrying out the activity. The significant objectives of yoga education are given below:

1.1. Awareness about health, hygiene and concentration.

1.2. Daily practice of postures (asanas), pranayama and meditation.

1.3. Healthy body along with improved concentration.

1.4. Development of intelligence-intellect.

1.5. Awareness of yogic diet and conduct leading to adoption of these disciplines in daily life.

1.6. Evaluation of self through family, society, nation and humanity at large.

1.7. Prayer and surrender unto the Lord should play an important role in life.

2. Achieving the Aims of Evaluation

2.1. In the common technique of evaluation, the attainment of an individual is compared with the average performance of the group. But in yoga education, the average or norm should not be suggested as the target performance of each individual. For example, the average time of a particular class while measuring deep breathing time cannot be the guiding factor for each child of the class. Every child should compete with one's previous performance and thus improve one's timing of any asana, trataka, pranayama and meditation.

2.2. Evaluation is used as a diagnostic tool also. The techniques of evaluation should be used that we may be able to locate the weak spots in the personality complex of an individual child, malfunctioning of any system or organ of the body, and imbalance in development. Yoga education should be so planned as to overcome the shortcomings and remove imbalances.

2.3. Subtle aspects of yoga imply subjective experiences. Evaluation of subjective experiences objectively is a very difficult task. The very fact that the experience is pleasant and refreshing works as a motivating force and inspires the Yoga practitioner to practise regularly, with faith. This motivation in due course becomes a determination.

2.4. Verbal information can be easily measured or evaluated. But this is only secondary aspect of yoga. Sadhaka may evaluate the behavioural aspect himself and improve conduct through self-evaluation.

2.5. Proportionate weightage should be given to physical, pranic, mental and intellectual aspects while planning evaluation in yoga education.

3.0 Evaluation Procedure

3.1. Evaluation of physical development should be based on due consideration of the indicators of good health. These indicators evaluate efficient functioning of the prominent systems of the body.

3.1(1) The first indicator shall not be comprised of only weight or only height. Ratio of weight and height is a more reliable indicator.

$$\frac{\text{Weight (Kilogram)}}{\text{Height (Centimeter)}} = 0.4 \text{ (norm)}$$

3.1(2) Instead of only weight, ratio of grip and weight is a better indicator.

3.1(3) The health of circulatory system is indicated by pulse rate per minute.

3.1(4) Generally, circumference of chest and abdomen are measured separately. But the ratio

$$\frac{\text{circumference of chest}}{\text{circumference of abdomen}}$$

greater than one indicated good health.

3.1(5) Elasticity of spine may be one of the indicators of the health of nervous system.

3.1(5.1) How long can one sit with spine erect.

3.1(5.2) Length of vertebral column in Paschimottan asan position length of vertebral column in the normal position–Elasticity of spine.

3.1(6) Two measures may be used for the respiratory system.

3.1(6.1) Circumference of chest with full breath-circumference after exhalation.

3.1(6.2) The time taken in seconds in exhalation during Bhramari pranayama or prolonged sound of Om.

3.1(7) In order to evaluate coordination of respiratory and circulatory systems, the following procedure may be adopted:

Pulse rate per minute after 50.meters race = (a).

Pulse rate per minute after 30 seconds = (b). b=a indicates good coordination of circulatory and respiratory system.

3.1(8) The measures for digestive system are; norms appetite, drinking 3-4 litres of liquid like water, milk juices and regular clearance of bowels.

3.1(9) In the assessment of excretory system besides normal excretion and urination, perspiration may also be considered. Information about these points may be collected through a questionnaire.

3.2 Evaluation of prana-shakti: Adolescents below 14 years are advised not to do retention of breath consequently besides 3.1.6.2 one more indicator may be used to evaluate discipline of prana shakti. This is average time of one breath in equalised breathing.

3.2(1) Pratyahara (introversion) dharna (concentration and meditation require to foundation of pranayama. Therefore, progress in savasana, yoganidra, trataka and meditation is indicative of discipline of prana.

3.3 Mental development is evaluated in terms of peace of mind, balance in emotions, and emotional disturbance does not leave permanent residue of tension.

3.3(1) Refreshing healthy sleep indicates that the mind is quiet and tension free.

3.3(1.1) Average time of daily sleep.

3.3(1.2) How long does it take to go to sleep?

3.3(1.3) Do you have to wait for long in order to go to sleep?

3.3(1.4) What is the theme of dreams if any?

3.3(2) Emotional development shall be evaluated in terms of personality adjustment with the help of psychological tests and inventories. These tools may very for linguistic and cultural variations.

3.4 Intellectual development is an aspect of Jnanamaya kosha. Achievement quotient in school subjects may be indicative of concentration, retention, analytical thinking and organisational ability.

Standardised psychological tests are available for intelligence.

3.4(1) Concentration influences speed of performance and correctness of the task done. Complexity of task may very according to the age group involved.

3.4(1.1) A printed sheet may be given to each child in the group. They may be asked to circle or cross a particular letter. Time given for the performance of the task is one minute. The number of correct letters circled or crossed is the score.

3.4(1.2) An example of a task from arithmetic may be. Take a number (say 3). Add. to it 3, 4, 5, repeatedly in sequence. Example of performance shall be 3, 6, 10, 15,18, 22, 27, 30, 34, 39..........

The score shall be number of correct additions done.

3.4(1.3) Similar exercise may be framed involving multiplication.

3.4(1.4) Numeral symbol test. A code is framed for conversion of numerals into symbols *e.g.*,

1	2	3	4	5	6	7	8	9	0
A	E	I	O	U	V	W	X	Y	Z

Numbers are to be written in the form of code or *vice versa*. 631, 735, 945, 832, as VIA, WIU, XOU--------------.

3.4(1.5) Letter–symbol test may be framed along the lines of 3.414.

3.4(2) Memory depends an concentration. If one does not concentrate on an impression, it is not retained even for a second. Expose or project a set of numerals, letters, words, or articles for a definite period say 5 to 10 seconds. The testees may be asked to write the objects exposed immediately. Memory score shall be the number of objects correctly remembered.

3.4(3) The abilities to make decisions and organise things or events are measured with the help of standardized tests for these purposes.

3.5 Spiritual development deals with the most subtle aspect of personality.

3.5(1) Values of life and ethical Values are the behavioral aspects of spiritual development. Bharateeya Shiksha Shodha Sansthan, Sarswati Kunj, Nirala Nagar, Lucknow, has published tools to evaluate values of life, ethical values and positive virtues.

3.5(2) Self concept is an important dimention of spiritual development. It is evaluated with the help of specially designed self concept inventories.

3.5(3) Story telling method may be used to assess assimilation of the code of conduct. A story pertaining to a yama or miyama is narrated. The group is asked to write the significant aspects of the story. The responses are evaluated to find out whether important behavioural points could be identified.

3.5(4) What is the place of meditation in daily routine? How long can one sit in meditation?

Subjective experiences during meditation may be recorded in the daily diary. The yoga teacher may use the diary in confidence to assess the progress of the pupil and to provide suitable guidance.

3.5(5) Self evaluation inventories in yoga education are available. One prepared by the author is given in the book (in Hindi). Yoga Shiksha kyon aur kaise, Vidya Bharati, gita school campus, Kurukshetra.

Yogic Methods and Techniques for Total Living

Hansa Jayadeva Yogendra

Man of the twentieth Century–on the threshold of the next millennium finds himself alienated from his moorings, cast adrift in the uncertain future, without a lodestar which can guide him to a determined goal of the 'greatest good of the greatest number'. But this seems to be receding like the horizon, notwithstanding the fantastic advances made in the field of science and technology; and more particularly the inroads made in the area of space exploration, inter-stellar travel on the one hand, and the other relating to the unchartered territory of the human brain, with its complex and complicated network of neurons, untouched glands and hormones which guard the secret of the Gods and the mystery of life on this planet.

If we are to survive the next century, then urgent and serious steps will have to be taken by the thinkers of the world–both in the East and the West–to chalk out a programme of sane living, guided by caring and sharing, irrespective of factors of caste, creed, colour, religion or national boundaries, which has fractured into pieces, this planet with its possibilities of establishing one government; tearing down the barriers which divides the East from the West.

The physical structure of man with its different systems held together by an indwelling spirit is in the danger of collapse, unless saner counsels prevail. We must stop abusing the 'outer shell' if the Spirit within is to be allowed free play. With this objective in mind, we, at the Yoga Institute, started a programme of health camps, in collaboration with medical fraternity, which is slowly recognising the validity and importance of Yoga at all levels, for ushering in a holistic approach to problems of life and living, confronting man all over the globe.

The Health Camps, initiated by the Yoga Institute–backed by professionals and experts in the field of mind, body and emotions, with its complicating inter-relatedness, are now being recognised by therapeutics of different views with their divergent emphasis and view points. Yoga is the only therapy which is concerned and cares for the Total Man, and not the fragmentary approach to deal with parts and not the whole. Yoga, hence is a Holistic approach for Total Health of the Total Man, body, mind and Spirit.

SCIENTIFIC RESULTS OF THE CAMP FOR DIABETICS

At a special camp for diabetics held at The Yoga Institute from 22nd to 28th July, 1987 some dramatic results were obtained. On the day that the camp commenced a sample of blood was collected at the Yoga Institute of the participating patients before and two hours after lunch. On the seventh day the same procedure was followed.

Below is seen the fasting and post-prandial results of the blood sugar.

Fasting Blood Sugar Values in mg./100 ml at the commencement and conclusion of the one week camp for diabetics held at The Yoga Institute in July 1987.

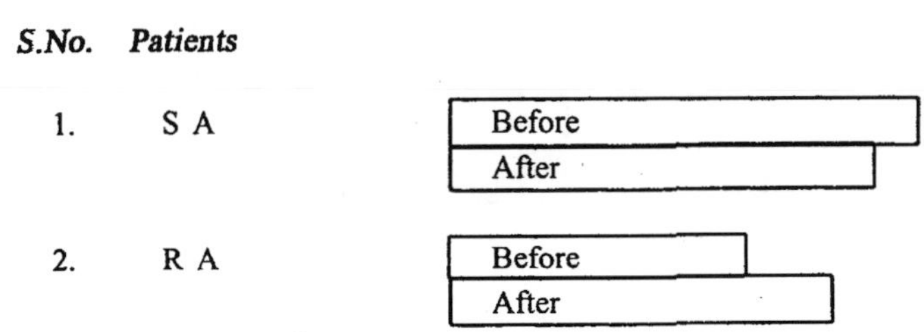

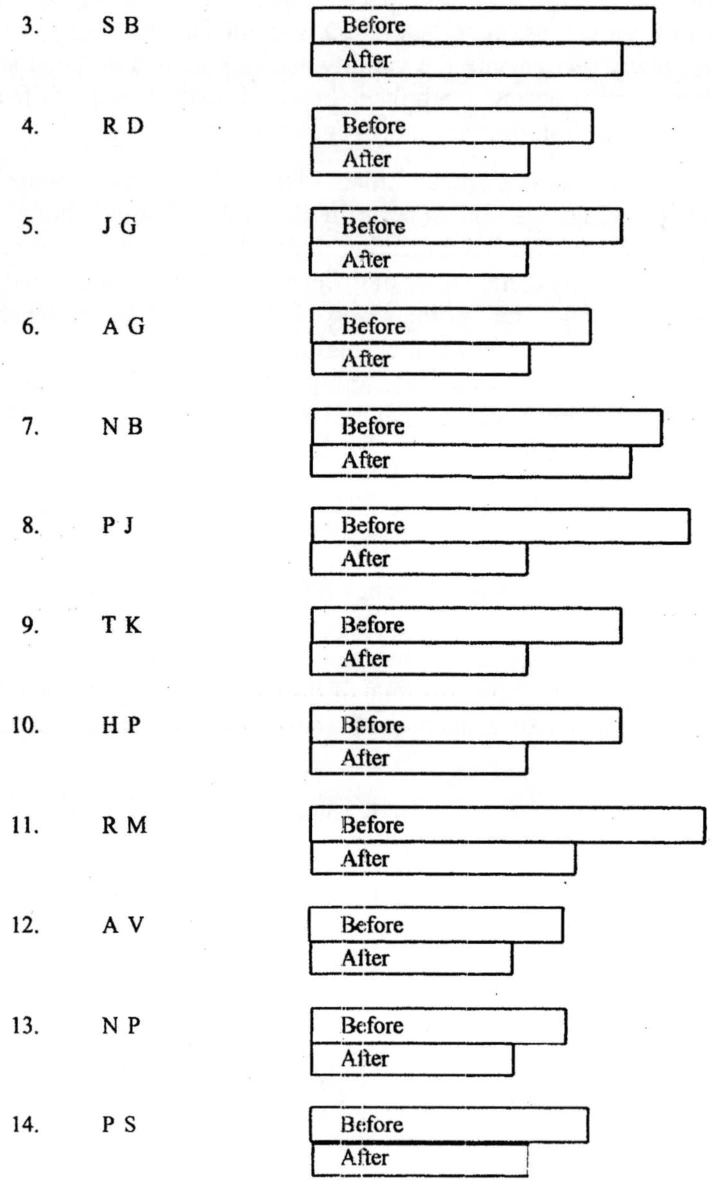
3. S B
Before
After
4. R D
Before
After
5. J G
Before
After
6. A G
Before
After
7. N B
Before
After
8. P J
Before
After
9. T K
Before
After
10. H P
Before
After
11. R M
Before
After
12. A V
Before
After
13. N P
Before
After
14. P S
Before
After

Post-prandial Blood Sugar Values in mg./100 ml at the commencement and conclusion of one week camp

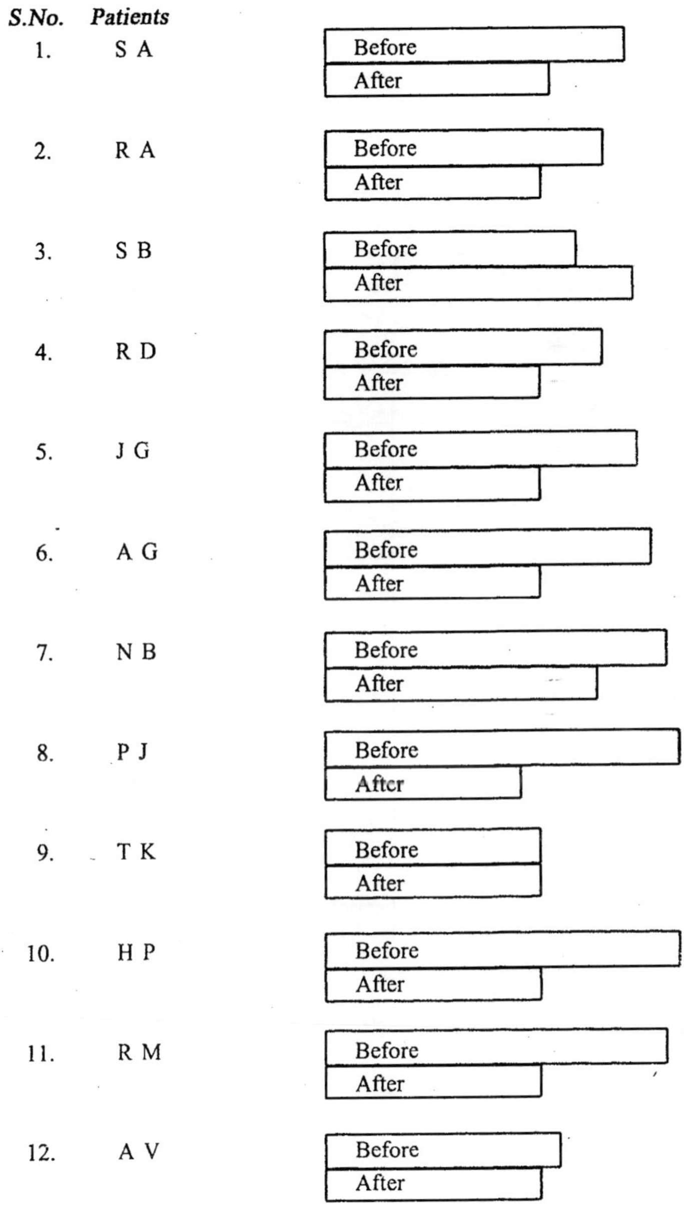

13. N P

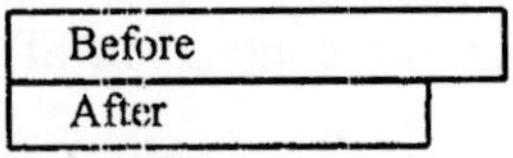

14. P S

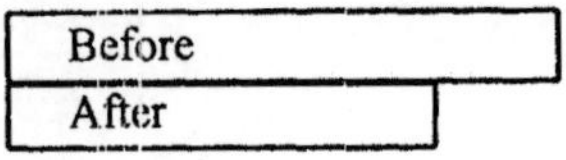

Note: SB and RA's readings were non-conclusive as they both had superimposed respiratory infection at that time.

Post-prandial Blood Sugar Value in mg./100 ml at the commencement and conclusion of one week Camp

S.No. Patients

1. S A

2. R A

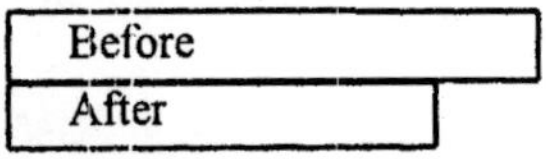

3. S B

4. R D

5. J G

6. A G

7. N B

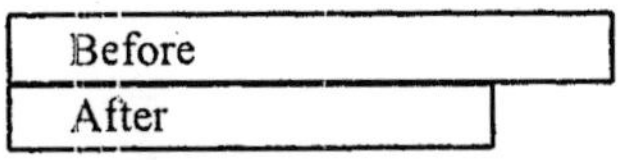

8. P J

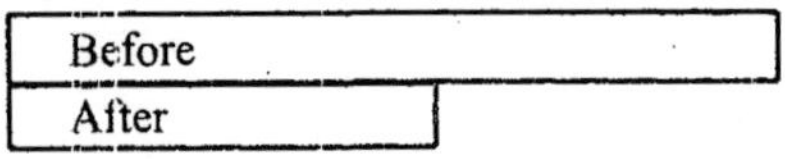

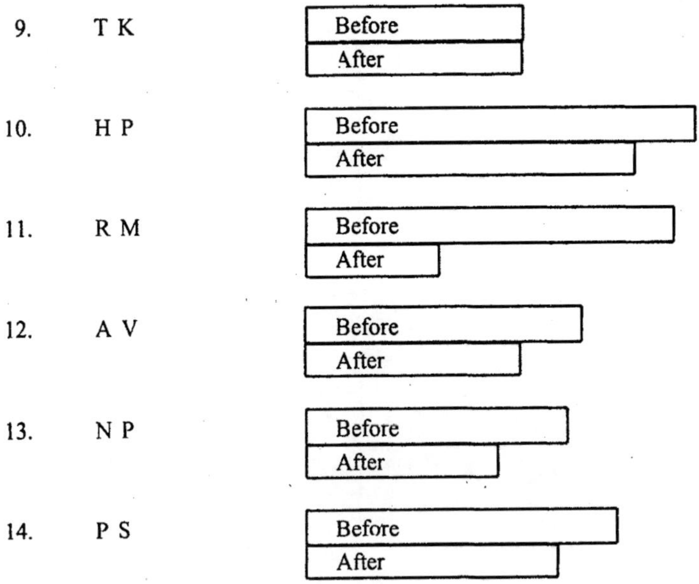

Note: SB and RA's readings were non-conclusive as they both had superimposed respiratory infection at that time.

Results of Health Camps held

Findings of the First Camp for Diabetics (1987)

Dr. V.S. Ajagaonkar assisted in the diabetes Yoga camp in 1987. When these camps were inaugurated, the book Yoga Therapy in Asthma, Diabetes and Heart Disease was published and principles, practices and scientific results were presented in this work. Reproduced below is the fasting blood sugar results at the commencement and conclusion of the camp.

S.No. Patients

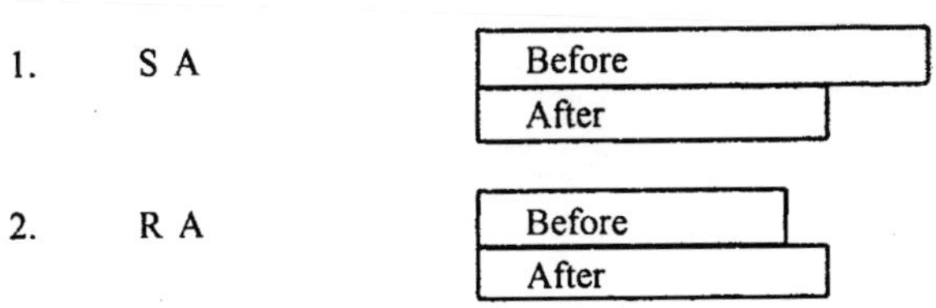

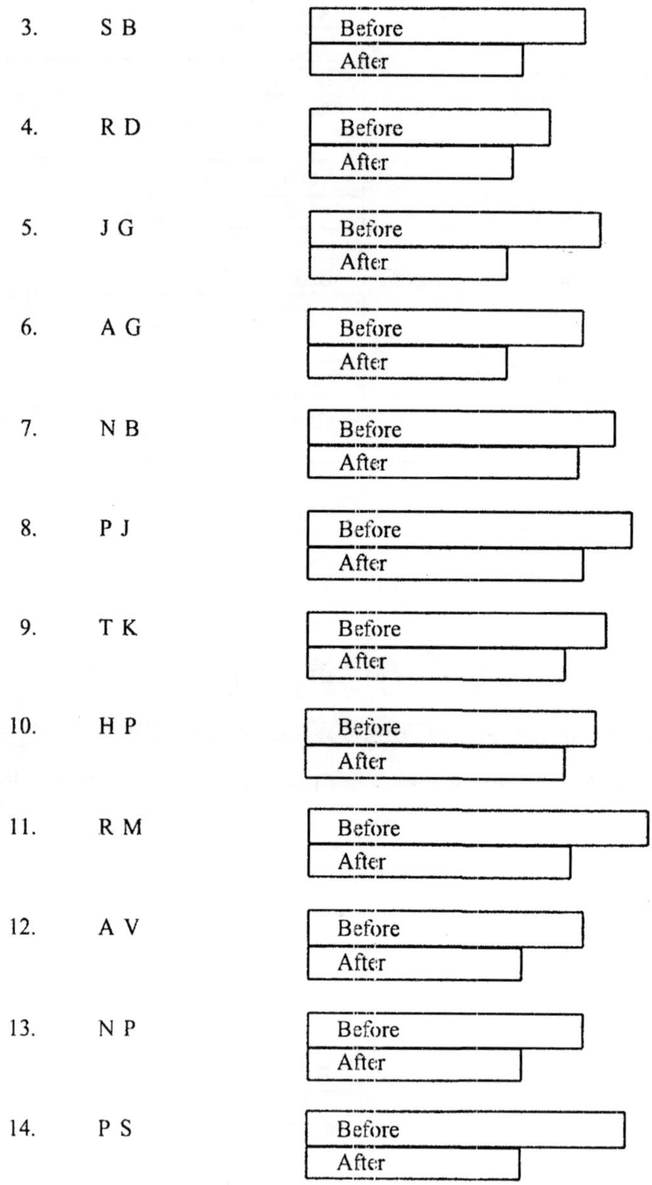
3. S B
Before
After
4. R D
Before
After
5. J G
Before
After
6. A G
Before
After
7. N B
Before
After
8. P J
Before
After
9. T K
Before
After
10. H P
Before
After
11. R M
Before
After
12. A V
Before
After
13. N P
Before
After
14. P S
Before
After

Benefits of the Coronary Care Camp

	Patients and their profiles at the time of joining camp	*Symptomatic Improvement (Subjective)*	*Objective Improvement assessed by Modern Test and procedures*	
			Electrocardio-graphy (ECG)	*Echocardiography (2 D Echo)**
1.	Male, 60 with MI and occasional HBP		Better	Better
2.	Male, 65 with MI, Angina & HBP	Yes	Same	Same
3.	Male, 58 with MI, Angina, HBP & Dia-B	-	Slight	
4.	Male, 58 with MI, Angina, HBP & Dia	Yes	-	Better
5.	Male, 63 with MI & HBP	Yes	Better	Better
6.	Male, 61 with MI, Angina & Diar-B	Slight	-	Slight
7.	Male, 69 with Angina	Yes	-	Same
8.	Male, 50 with MI and Angina	Yes	-	Better
9.	Male, 57 with MI, occasional HBP & Dia-B	-	Same	
10.	Female, 50 with Angina & HBP	Yes	Better	Same

Note * 2 D Echocardiography checks the health of heart's wall and heart's values by using ultra sound waves.

KEY

DIA=Diabetes

Dia B=Borderline Diabetes

M.I.=Myocardial Infarction Damaged Heart following Coronary Artery Disease

H.B.P.=High Blood Pressure (Hypertension)

Group of Diabetics Who Improved

FBS–Fasting Blood Sugar Reading

PP–Post Prandial Reading

PAT–Patients

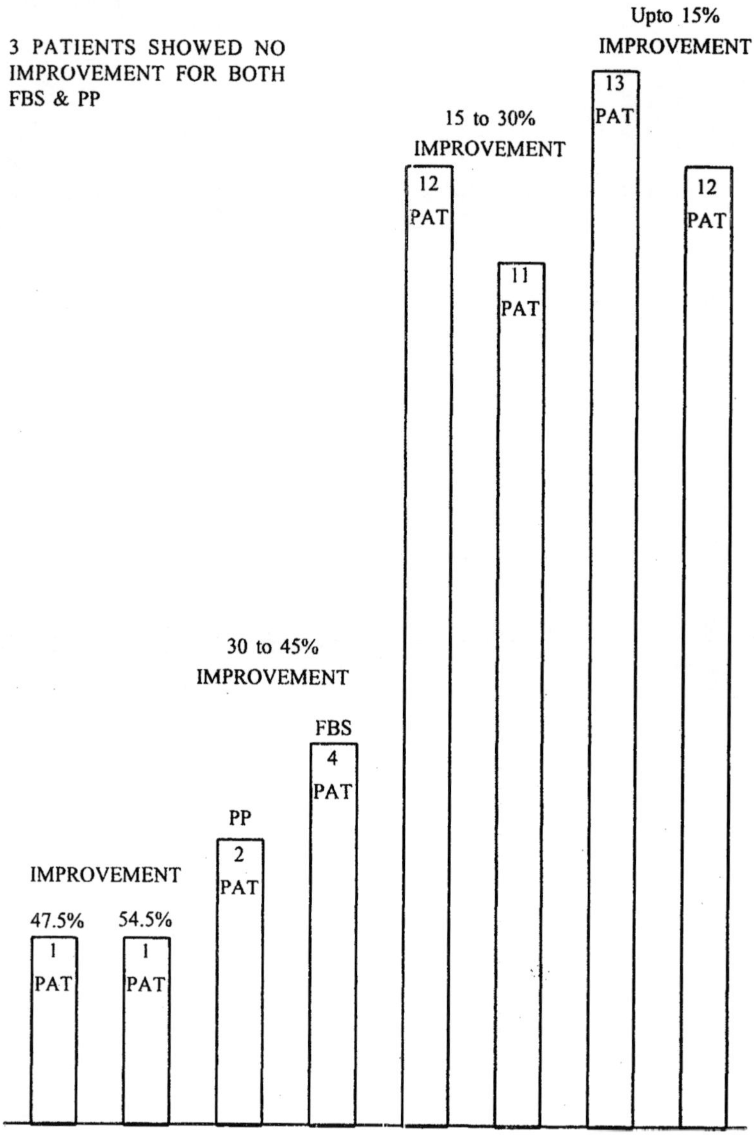

Tension-free states

This category includes feelings of contentment, peace, tranquility a happy frame of mind. 54% of the individuals reported feeling this way all the time, 28% felt this way most of the time. 15% felt this way sometimes and 3% reported feeling this way rarely.

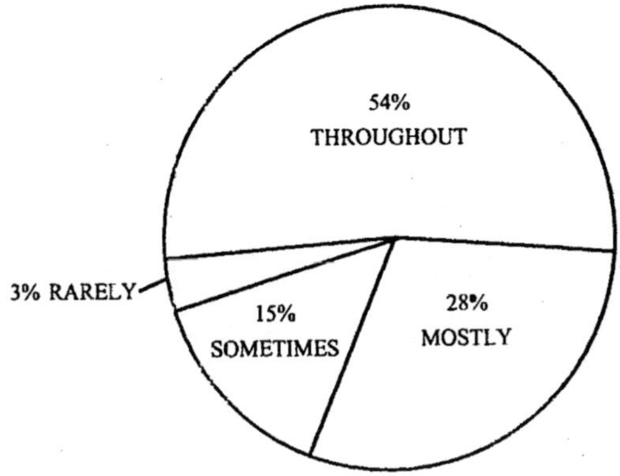

Attitude Changes

50% individuals reported a positive attitude change which means that their outlook to life is healthier. It is more positive. They have become more accepting and are able to handle the disease better, more constructively. 15% reported a bit of change. 33% reported no change and 2% felt a worsening effect.

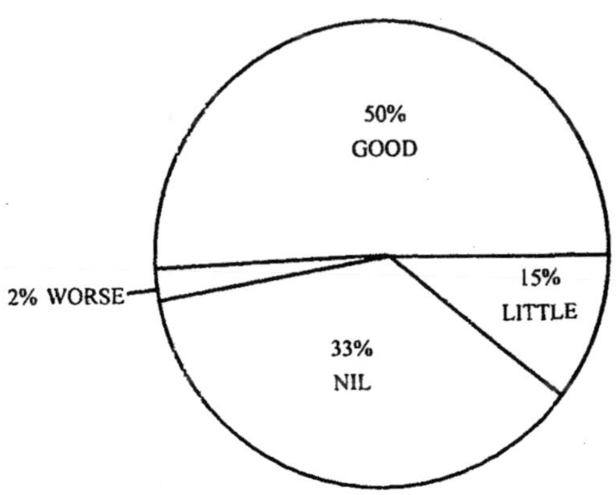

Improvement over earlier Negative States

This relates to feelings of anxiety, tension, hostility, anger, worry etc. Such feelings were rare in 37% of the individuals, 44% reported that they were present sometimes 5% reported having them frequently and 14% had these feelings often.

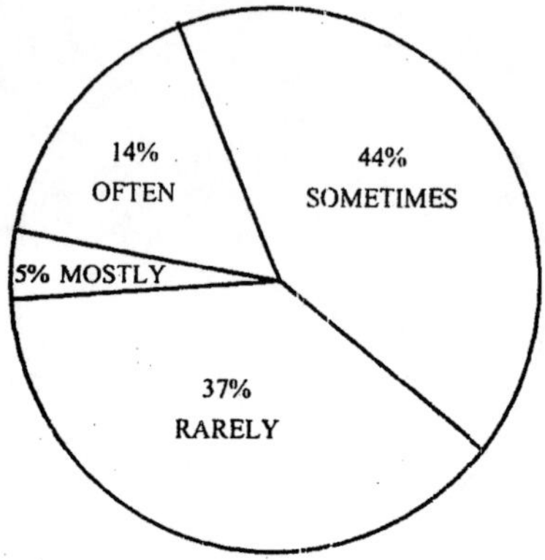

Improvement in Physical Feeling

52% of the campers reported that they were feeling physically good at this point of time. 31% reported that they were feeling physically good at this point of time. 31% reported that they were feeling physically uneasy and 17% reported that they were definitely better since the start of the camp.

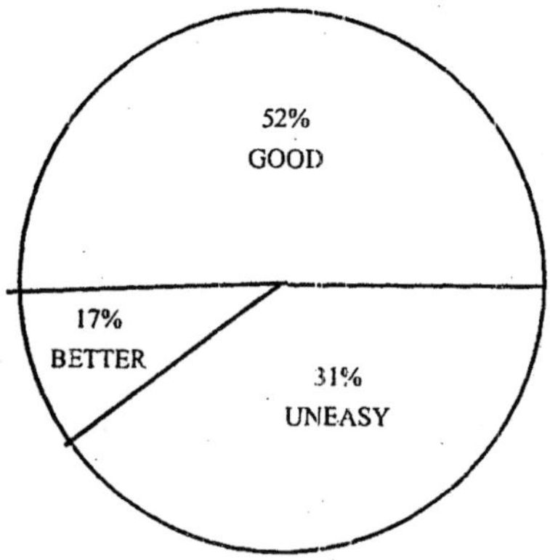

Follow up period	*No. of patients*
2 months	4
6 months to 1 year	10
1 to 2 years	29
2 to 3 years	1
3 to 4 years	5
	49

Serum Cholesterol level	*Number of patients*	
(mg.%)	*Before*	*After*
200 mg./or less	25	32
201 to 240	16	16
241 to 265	3	1
266 or more	5	0

Serum Triglyceride	*Number of patients*	
(mg.%)	*Before*	*After*
100 or less	7	17
101 to 160	21	27
161 to 300	19	5
301 or more	2	0

Serum HDL Cholesterol Level	*Number of patients*	
(mg.%)	*Before*	*After*
45 or less	26	6
46-55	16	19
56 or more	7	24

Special Camps Conducted at the Yoga Institute in 1987 as part of the 70 year celebrations

Coronary care camp	*Airway camp for asthmatics*	*Camp for diabetics*	*ENT Problems*	*Gastro-intentional Problems*
May	*June*	*July*	*August*	*September*
15	26	16	5	18

Unhealthy Habits

A staggering 87% of the individuals had modified their life style and given up smoking, drinking and a sedentary life-style. 13% reported that they still had some unhealthy habits. One of the participants seemed to echo most of them when he said, We have realized that life is for living–and we live each day fully, joyously and with faith–"

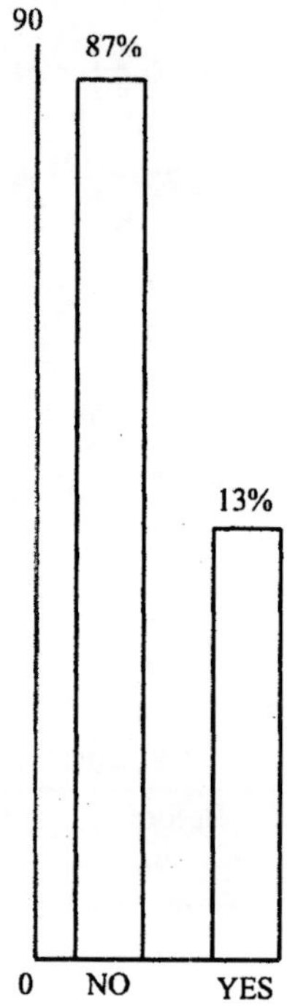

Decline in Urine Sugar as tested by 'Diastrix'
(taking into account the highest reading for the day)

Patients	*SA*	*CSM*	*HRP*	*SR*	*MS*	*ADV*	*NP*	*PS*	*RA*	*SB*	*RD*	*JGG*	*G*	*NII*	*PPJ*	*TK*
Day 1	N	N	***	****	N	N	N	N	N	*	N	N	N	***	***	Tr
Day 1	N	N	**	***	N	N	N	N	N	N	N	N	N	**	Tr	N
Day 7	N	N	Tr	N	N	N	N	N	N	N	N	N	-	*	Tr	N

N–Normal
Tr–Trace
- –Reading not taken

Date	*Blood Pressure*	*Triglycerides*	*Cholesterol*	*Remarks*
11.1.80	180/110	315 mg	285 mg	First detected
21.8.80	130/90	140 mg	252 mg	Under cover of drugs
3.4.82	130/90	190 mg	270 mg	Under Yoga; no drugs
1.9.82	120/80	150 mg	240 mg	Advanced Yoga; no drugs

Need and Scope of Applied Research in Yoga for Physical Education and Sports

Narain Prakash

The Purpose and Functions of Research

Research has proved to be an essential tool in leading man towards progress, hence it is vital for every type of development reducing man's areas of ignorance by discovering new truths, which in turn lead to better predictions, better methods of doing things and better products.

Scope of Applied Research in Yoga

"The entire range of muscular activity from 0 to 100% is rightly the providence of physical education" says Stien, Hause (1964). These remarks show that yogic practices deserve rightful place in the armamentarium of physical education that they occupy today. It would be a matter of greater significance if their contribution to motor skill learning process of other physical activities and to the mental fitness of the high performance athletes could be recognised and harnessed in the national interests as is being done by a number countries abroad so much so that ability to relax, which is the main feature of all yogic practices, has been included as one of the items of the battery of fitness evaluation (Miller, 1986). Therefore, to write on "research in Yoga" for promotion of research, innovation and evaluation in physical education will not be a matter of surprise to anybody as yoga has not only been recognised as an integral part of education but of physical education and sports as well (Kothari Commission Report, 1964-66; National Policy on Education 1986 and revised in 1992). Research in physical education and sports if it be considered worthwhile, requires not only the knowledge of the methods and techniques suited to the field but also an understanding of the significant problems that need to tackled, may these be immediate or of long tenure, by all means–indigenous or borrowed. Besides, the research programmes and research techniques also have to fit in with the genious, the philosophical, social and cultural background of the country and her educational system.

It has repeatedly been stressed that yoga should be propogated and widely practised and included in the school syllabus as an alternative form of physical education. (Draft-National Sports Policy–1979). Nay, the possibility of yoga practices to be utilized for improving the stamina and physical efficiency of sportsmen with a view to improving the sports standards should also be explored–has been further emphasised. But alas! nothing substantial has been achieved except the inclusion of yogic practices in the syllabus of schools. The reasons are not too far to seek. The people responsible for implementing the scheme are not yoga-oriented as neither they have learnt and practiced nor have indepth study of the literature on the subject. In addition to their disinterestedness because of the reasons mentioned above the national coaches of different sport disciplines seem to have their own personal whims and doubts and baseless reservations to include yogic practices in training scheduled of their athletes.

Research in the field of physical education and sports needs to be identified with a better understanding of the individual athlete in terms of his needs, interests, attitudes, potentialities and limitations as well; a better understanding training/teaching-learning process and the conditions under which it is most carefully carried on; better selection for members of team for a competition and training and more suitable choice of the activity matching an individual's personality; better means of maintenance of fitness during off season; better methods of training and conditioning; better policies for development of sports in general and for the care of athletes in particular; better techniques and implements of evaluation the progress of the athletes in the status of his health and fitness skill and performance.

Application of Yogic Practices in the Field of Physical Education and Sports

Yoga, in its technical sense, is supposed to deal primevally with spiritual unfoldment of the individual. Hence, really speaking neither physical education nor sports are directly the fields of yoga in its proper sense. However, it has necessarily to do with health and fitness related aspects of body and mind which are deemed essential even for the success in one's endeavours in any sphere of life. Ayurveda--the ancient science of Indian medicine and yoga consider positive health to be the foremost and essential prerequisite for success in all sorts of efforts, ranging from materialistic gains (worldly pleasures) of lowest category to that of self-realization (Vidyalankar, 1944). The word "Yoga" actually signifies functional integration at highest level of spirituo-psycho-somatic development ensuring not only the health of body but also experiencing the sense of well-being of the senses, the mind and the soul simultaneously (Shastri, 1954). It has, therefore, laid down certain ways and means in the form of various physical and mental (Somato-phychic and psychosomatic) procedures to counteract the malicious environmental influences possible from within and without the organism.

It is apparently clear from the scheme of yoga practices laid down in ancient yogic texts, the all such yoga practices including yamas–the rules of social hygiene; Niyama the rules of personal hygiene; Asanas–the postural patterns; Pranayamas–the breathing exercises; Meditation etc. are prescribed to prepare the aspirant progressively for higher practice of yoga proper under supervised guidance. These preparatory practices seem to be designed with purpose of conditioning and/or reconditioning/ deconditioning the body-mind machinery so as to extend its range of adaptability (Vinekar, 1967). Then, under the concept explained above, what could be expected of yoga to play a significant role in the fields of physical education and sports, is basic question. The answer goes in favour of the yogic practices as many of the problems that the people are facing today in the areas of health and fitness, medicine, education and competitive sports. Teachers of physical education and sports or trainers in an educational institution are responsible for planning and implementation of programmes for "Health for all" including normal exceptional (too weak or excellent), retarded, handicapped, deformed and disabled and rehabilitation programme for those who rejoin after illness or injury alongwith preparing the potentially talented athletes to excel keeping in view the availability of facilities and finances. Thus the areas can be broadly classified into two–(1) Health and fitness for all, (2) Excellence in competitive sports.

(1) Health and Fitness–The dynamic development of modern science and technology and the achievements of contemporary civilization have brought about social and economical transformations so rapidly and to such a scale that there is every danger to the ecological balance of man bringing about an unprecedented increase in his health problems including low resistance to stress and disease, birth of a large number of psychosomatic diseases etc. The situation has made very much imperative for the physical educationists to find out suitable programmes of physical activities for our health problems to keep up with events as rapidly as the world in which we operate and to counteract the influences impinged upon by the environmental conditions in view of proper protection (preventive aspect) maintenance and promotion of general health and fitness of the people for effective and qualitative living and productivity.

(2) Excellence in Sports–The recent trend to prove the physical superiority of the nation and to show its worth in the international field of games and sports and hence establish its supremacy has thrown a challenge to the physical educationists, the coaches and their co-workers in ancilliary disciplines to find out such phenomenal and procedural (ergogenic) aids that might prove to be helpful in excelling in competitive sports.

Therefore, the rising enthusiasm for sports and physical activity, may it be meant for health and physical fitness for effective living or an effort in the direction of achieving top level performance in a competitive sport, must lead constantly to expand interest of all concerned in the scientific research related to bio-physiological changes from various forms of physical activities or practices including yoga. There are a number of references available in ancient yoga texts regarding the beneficial effects of yogic practices that accure from the regular practices of yogic techniques. Among these traditional claims–some are ordinary, while a few seem to be extraordinary or exceptional. Then, there are present-day scientists of 20th century who have unvield a number of physical, mental, emotional, physio-chemical and neurological factors that are beneficially influenced by yoga practices. The results of such scientific studies can be taken to be advantageous to almost all spheres of life. However, the scope is limited here to the application of yogic practices in the fields of education and physical education only. Let us first have a view of how far the various aspects of education and physical education have been delt with–in some selected research studies. Then only, it would be possible to suggest scope and nature of applied yoga research to be taken further for its integration into education and physical education.

The studies by Raseh (1958), De Vries (1962), Giri (1964), Dhanraj (1974), Kanade and Gharote (1990), Ganguly and Gharote (1974), Romano Waski and Parek (1970) show that yogic practices have favourable effects upon the important components of physical fitness, especially on flexibility and cardiovascular efficiency. The studies of Gharote (1971), Green and Green (1971, 1973), Kocher (1972, 76), Kochar and Pratap (1972), Pratap (1968), show that both short term as well as long term practice of yoga substantially improves the emotional stability, steadiness, immediate memory and alleviates anxiety, hostility, neuroticism etc. which gives a ray of hope in having a measure for minimizing the deliquency and unrest among our youth. The relaxation procedures of yoga have also been found helpful in early recovery from fatigue (Mall, Chaudhary and Giri (1977), Rathbone (1969). Physiological and biochemical studies conducted on normal, healthy as well as sick adults and simile people of both the sexes have shown favourable effects upon parameters like oxygen consumption, carbondioxide elimination, rate and depth of respiration, arterial blood pressure and acidity; blood lactate, blood sugar and blood cholestrol level; heart rate, flow and distribution of blood; excretion of pepsin and sugar in urine; salivary secretion; skin resistance reaction time; muscle tone; reetal, skin and sublinguil temperature; EEG pattern, perception, personality and affective behaviour (Abosi, 1974; Bhole, 1988, 1990; Wallace, 1970; Swami Kuvalyananda and Vinekar, 1963; Karambelkar, 1969; Datey and *et al.*, 1983).

In view of the favourable effects of yogic practices on human organism, the modern scientists presume that yogic practices bring about higher and higher conditioning of limbic system which is thought to be responsible for regulation of autonomic and endocrinal functions and the affective behaviour by virtue of which the practicant gets greater and greater volitional control over them leading to recovery from homeostatic dysfunction in the case of sick and towards perfection of biological equilibrium in the case of normal person (Anand *et al.*, 1961; Wenger and Bagchi, 1961).

Preliminary Steps for Applied Research

Establishment of Regional Research and Training Institutes of Yoga–The studies so far conducted to evaluate the effects of yogic practices on the status of health and physical fitness included a very small number of subjects. Further, no comparative study of two types of programmes *i.e.* yoga and any other system of physical activity has been made. Similarly, no comparative study has been made on male and female subjects. Studies conducted to gauge psychological and physio-biochemical effects are no exception to such luconas as mentioned above. However, replication of studies in most of the investigations made by medicose and other scientists in India and abroad has proved beyond doubt that yogic practices help in developing and maintenance of better biological integration than any other conventional system of physical activity.

In order to overcome such drawbacks and to further verify the beneficial effects of yogic practices it would be in fitness of thing if Govt. of India could establish six or so regional research institutions of yoga each one with one school and one college attached and run only on lines of yogic way of life.

Personnel Management in Research Institutes of Yoga–The dearth of adequate competent personnel to man the research institutes/departments of yoga is only matched today by the lack of vision, background of language and literature, personal practice of and experience in yoga, originality, and even of elementary knowledge of latest research techniques. However, only a few are trying to fill the void. What to say of an army of private yoga institutions, some of our government/government aided institutes are headed and sub-ordinated by such psueds personnel and hence the outcome, if it cannot be said nil, it is definitely below expectation. Therefore, Govt. should see that the heads of such institutions are highly qualified in the science of yoga. The director/head should be one who is most effective, stimulative, and continuously active in research. He should be most prone to have thorough knowledge of and insight into his field. As yoga is behavioural science, he should be assisted by specialists from other allied disciplines like philosophy and literature, Anatomy, physiology, biochemistry, biophysics, anthropometry, human biology, psychology, education nutrition, sociology etc.

Further, research in yoga needs cooperation and mutual understanding between the various agencies like health, medicine, education and sports, industry, defence etc. in conducting various projects. A better communication between such agencies can be developed by organising symposia etc.

Production of Yoga Literature in National and Regional Languages–The major problem being faced in wide popularization of yogic practices is that the original yoga text books are in Sanskrit language and these are neither being read nor interpreted properly by the common man in general and scientists in particular. The task of translation and interpretation needs to be taken up immediately by the joint groups of scholars from the fields of yoga literature, yoga philosophy, regional languages and sciences well-versed in Sanskrit language. Further, there is need of popular yoga series to be available in all regional languages with elaborate illustrations and instructions to meet the demands of the masses across the whole country. No less important is the job of writing of books for each class of the school and college going population. N.C.E.R.T. must take up the challenge and with the help of qualified people from all over the country should complete the task as early as possible. It would be very much appreciated if N.C.E.R.T. establishes its separates wing of yoga quarterly journal exclusive for yoga to keep the teachers in schools and colleges abreast of the latest developments and innovations made in the fields of yoga and applied sciences.

Aquisition of and Training in Monitorying of Sophisticated Research Equipments–Modern era is that of science and technology. Any scientific research, particularly yoga, needs sophisticated instruments and their expertise use. Govt. of India must ensure that selected yoga Institutes/departments are equipped with the latest equipments needed to evaluate subtle psychophysiological effects of yogic practices. If need be, some suitable people should be sent abroad to tour developed countries to locate latest technology and gadgets and also to have training in their handling and monitorying. Later on such instrument can improvised and/or manufactured locally.

Standardization of Procedures and Nomenclature of Yogic Practices–It has been observed that there exist variations in the procedures of performing asanas or any other practice from expert to expert and place to place. Besides, the Asanas are practiced in variety of rhythms *i.e.*, in slow and fast sequence. Some time one and the same yogic practice is known by different names. Therefore, there is an urgent need of standardization of performing technique and their nomenclature at national level so that research projects could be conducted and their results could also be composed and verified to draw rational conclusions. Such a project could be entrusted by the ministry of Human Resource Development to a committee comprising of experts drawn from different corners of the country.

Estimation of Energy Expenditure of Yogic Practices– Estimation of energy expenditure in each of the yogic practice separately and therefore to calculate total energy expenditure after undergoing one of the progressive tables of practices to be performed daily as a part of general routine, is the need of the day. This could give us an idea as how much an individual has to exert to maintain one's minimum fitness level and as such graded tables of practices could be developed for different age, sex and vocational group.

Research Regarding the Indications and Contraindications– There are no definite indications or contraindications available supported by scientific evidences for the prescription of particular yogic practice either for different age and sex groups or for people suffering from different ailments. Hence, scientific research institutes of yoga should be asked to do the needful within stipulated time and conclusion drawn by holding symposium. Such project could taken by the Ministry of Health which is responsible for "Health for all" scheme.

Simplification of Definitions and Important Yoga Concepts– Different definitions and important concepts of yoga should be so simplified and graded through research as are easily operable and understandable at different educational levels so that their application in different spheres of later life could easily be made possible by every one.

Yoga and Physical Education and Sports

Yoga as an alternate form of Physical Education–Yoga can ensure larger participation as health-activity under "Health for all" scheme because most of the students do not participate in vigorous physical activities like games and sports or their parents do not allow their wards or the school/college has no provision of facilities because any of the following reasons:

(a) There is always risk of temporary or permanent injury which an zeopardize or hamper their studies which are dearer to them than play.

(b) A notion has been developed in the minds of the people that participation in vigorous physical activities makes the children disinterested in their studies.

(c) Another notion that has found prominent is that participation in vigorous physical activities needs rich nutritious diet which is out of reach of common people.

(d) Most of the games need costly equipment/uniform which every parent cannot provide.

(e) Most of the modern sports need spacious playfield for which most of the schools/colleges have no provision.

Application of Research Results–Moreover, it is unfortunate that the results of yogic research shown by number of enthusiasts in India and abroad are neither applied by the Indian educationists including physical educationists nor by the medicos in the existing practices for the benefit of our masses.

Sports Authorities Need Understanding of Yoga–It has been observed that our institutions like sports authority of India, National Institute of Sports and National Federations in different sport-disciplines have developed a sort of monopoly over our sportsmen and their representatives hardly allow/offer anybody else to evaluate either the effects of some better techniques like yoga or the biotypological characteristics of our top athletes. They neither do such useful work themselves nor allow others, even if there is no interference in their regular work-outs. In case we are all interested in improving the existing standards in the field of physical education and sports we will have to create a befitting and congenial atmosphere to perform the task of applied research as far as yoga is concerned.

Who should Teach Yoga in Schools and Colleges?–There is controversy as who should take up the teaching of yoga in schools and colleges. Today this responsibility lies mostly with physical education teachers. It has been observed that the physical education teachers being of extrovert nature cannot justify achieving goods as desired. Their behaviour is goal oriented which is outside the body while yogic practices are of internal and introspective nature. Therefore, it is suggested that teachers from other disciplines who have an aptitude of yoga should be oriented in the subject and be entrusted with the job otherwise also the teachers of physical education are already overloaded with the responsibility of training/coaching various teams for regular competitions through out the year.

Blending of modern sport technology with ancient discipline of Yoga: "Sports, music and dance are perhaps the closest discipline to meditative training" Qpine Joel and Levly (1985). They further point out that peak performance in performance arts, like the above, related to the naturally blissful, energised, creative, and peaceful experience of the quiet and concentrated mind. Hence, there is every possibility that yogic practices could likely accelerate the pace of such experiences mentioned above leading nearer to the peak performance (designated a sort of "flow state" by the performers). Physical education teachers and coaches should expect that judicious blending of modern sports technologies and ancient disciplines of yoga particularly for mental fitness training of talented athletes might prove rewarding in an endeavour to win pride of place in international arena (Gharote, 1990). How the two could be blended depends, how the sports-scientists and yoga-scientists communicate mutually and understand each other's points of views and decide the line of action for indepth research as is being done in other countries.

Development of minimum physical tests and progressive Yoga-practice tables: On the part of physical educationists, there is need to develop minimum physical fitness standards for different age, sex and vocational groups. Once these are developed and standardized, separate tables of graded yogic practices could be put to test if these could fulfill minimum needs through out life.

Integration of yoga into learning of sports: Logical analysis and standardization of the different stages of each individual yoga practice is essential for proper skill development and perfection in the same. Simultaneously there is also need to find out through latest technology of myography as which muscles/muscle-groups are actively involved in the execution of each yogic practice and also those which are needed to be relaxed. In case a child can learn such things at an early stage, he/she can apply this knowledge while learning the motor skills of other physical activities.

Relationship between relaxation and motor skill learning and aquisition: Whether, it is a matter of successful participation or that of excellence in games and sports, motor-skill learning and aquisition is an important factor. At the same time, it is a well known fact that a relaxed state is a critical component of grasping and learning process. If that is the case, then yogic practice can definitely play a significant role as most of them relaxation inducing and tension reducing techniques. Therefore, it needs to be probed if children who practice yoga for at least three months or more could learn selected motor-skills earlier and better than those of the control group. Similarly, studies could be conducted if learning of some fine arts like music, dance, drama, painting including handwriting, sculpturing could be facilited through yoga-practice (Coville-1979).

Discriminative relaxation and development of athletic skills: In yogic practices, more particularly in Asanas, the skill of discriminative relaxation is developed as it is emphasised that the antagonistic muscles should be kept relaxed while maintaining a particular postural pattern. This is stressed with the principle in mind that the muscle-activity is controlled in such a way that muscles not specifically required for the task are quiet, and those which are required are fired at the minimum level to save energy. Investigations need to be conducted if the discriminative relaxation skill achieved through yoga-practices could be successfully integrated into learning and developing athletic skills and ratio application found beneficially influential even while actually fighting the competition.

Relationship between self-control-self-regulation and postponement of fatigue and early recovery: It is a well known fact that consistent practices of yoga develops the skill of self-control and self-regulation progressively over the mind-body complex. Hence, comparative studies comprising of practitioners and non practitioners of yoga need to undertaken to find out if fatigue does not set in yoga-practitioner comparatively at an early, if a definite task is done over a period of time and also to gauge the period of recovery in both the cases so as to verify the efficacy of yogic practices in postponing fatigue and an early recovery–an indication of fitness level achieved. This may further likely encourage to find out the effectiveness of yoga practices on an individual's productivity level also in any sphere.

Prevention and correction of postural deformities through yoga: Some weak, overworked and habitually tense children develop or have a tendency to develop certain postural deformities. It needs to investigated if such deformities could be prevented and/or corrected through regular practice of some appropriate asanas where in emphasis is laid upon systematic stretching and contracting of skeletal-muscles and thereby strengthening them so as to keep the muscles intact with the bones to which they are attached.

Prevention and care of sport-injuries through yoga: Sport persons have a tendency to get some of their particular muscles shortened because of constant use of certain muscle groups in a peculiar was in different games/sports and hense become prone to pulls and strains and rupture in some cases. Such injuries can be prevented by the practice of asanas wherein passive and steady stretching is emphasised progressively. Therefore, asanas could form part of the warming up and conditioning programme. Similarly, such procedures could be useful in the treatment and rehabilitation of muscular injuries like spasm etc. It has also been observed that practice of asanas prevents and gives relief from muscular distress/soreness caused by too much indulging in vigorous physical activities (De Vries, 1962), Bury (1971) has also suggested the utility of asanas in the prevention of accidents and injuries.

Regulation of and Control Over Alternate Breathing Cycles: Alternate breathing cycles the shifting of which takes place after about one and half an hour with a short gap when one breathes through both the nostrils, most likely mirror shifts in brain function from one hemisphere to the other while breathing through both the nostrils shows most balanced state of mind, brain and body which allows an integration of rational and intiative, detailed and global functions associated with the two hemispheres of the brain (Saraswati, 1994). During this period, it seems, the information flows more smoothly across the Corpus collosum–a bundle of brain fibers that forms the communication link between two sides of the brain. The truth behind these concepts of swar-yoga needs to be verified experimentally if variations in performance are found under different patterns of breathing as contemplated by ancient

Indian seers. The effectiveness of breathing patterns computability in scheduling the timings of meals, rest and training in additional investigations with cooperation neurophysiologists and biochemists of medical sciences.

Tackling of Deliquency and Indiscipline Through Yoga: Yogic practices are known for quietening somatic muscle activity which is accompanied by a domination in the state of excitability in the sympathetic division of the hypothalamus. With the consistent practice one learn to consciously minimize those mental and physical states that decrease and impair one's effectiveness and to increase those that enhance one's performance. Such training provides key to self-regulation and self-control in one's conduct and the changed life style. Longitudinal studies need to be undertaken to know if consistent practice could make the practicants more sensitive and earning reflecting their patience perseverance, tolerance and other moral qualities in their behaviour. This could, perhaps, help tackling of the rising problems of deliquency and indiscipline in educational institutions for which Psudo–sportspersons are generally held responsible.

References

1. Abosi, S. and Bohus, B. (1973), "Training for oxygen shortage," Jour. of technical track & field athletics, 51:124-1629.
2. Acarya Susruta (1954), "Translated by Kaviraj Dr. Ambika Dutta Shastri, Chaukhambha Sanskrit Series, Varanasi-1.
3. Anand, B.K. and *et al* (1961), "Studies on Shri Ramananda Yogi during his stay in an air tight box, Ind. Jour. Med. Res., 49:82-89.
4. Bhole, M.V. (1988), "Physiological benefits through yoga," Yoga Mimamsa, Vol. XXVII, No. 1 to 2, 119-127.
5. Bhole, M.V. (1990), "Stress management for executives and yoga," Yoga Mimamsa, Vol. XXIX, No. 1, 49-55.
6. Bury, H.C. (1971), "Athletic fitness: Its role in prevention accidents and injuries," Practitioner 206:227-233.
7. Coville, C.A. (1979) "Relaxation in physical education curricula," The physical educator, Vol. 36. No.-4.
8. Datey, K.K., Gharote, M.L. and Pavri, S. (1983), "Yoga and your heart," JAICO Publishing House, Bombay.
9. De Vries, H.A. (1961), "Prevention of muscular distress after exercise," Res. Quarterly, 32:177-185.

10. De Vries, H.A. (1962), "Evaluation of static stretching procedures for improvement of flexibility, Res. Quart. 33:2:222-229.
11. Dhanraj, V.H. (1974), "The effects of yoga and the 5 BX fitness plan on selected physiological parameters, Ph.D. Thesis, University of Alberta, Canada.
12. Ganguly, S.K. and Gharote, M.L. (1974) ,"Cardiovascular efficiency before and after yogic training," Yoga Mimamsa, Vol. XVII; No. 1, 89-97.
13. Giri, C. (1963), "Yoga and physical fitness with special reference to athletics," A research report submitted to the Govt. of India through K.S.M.Y.M. Samiti, Lonavla.
14. Gharote, M.L. (1973), "Effect of yogic training on physical fitness," Yoga Mimamsa, 15:4:31-35.
15. Gharote, M.L. (1988), "Yoga and sports," Yoga Mimamsa, Vol. XXVII, No. 1 & 2, 94-107.
16. Gharote, M.L. (1990), "Applied Yoga," Kaivalyadhama S.M.Y.M., Samiti, Lonavla.
17. Green, E.E. and Green, A.M. (1971), "On the meaning of transpersonal: some metaphysical perspectives, J. Transpers. Psychol., 3-27-46.
18. Green E.L. and Green, A.M. (1973), "Volition as metaforce in the field of mind theory, Voluntary controls programme research Deptt., The Menninger Foundation, U.S.A.
19. Kanade, V.K. and Gharote, M.L. (1990) ,"Effects of yogic training on physical fitness and selected athletic events, Yoga Mimamsa, Vol. XXIX, No. 1, 55-66.
20. Karambelkar *et al* (1969), "Effect of yogic asanas on uropepsin excretion," Ind. Jour. Med. Res. 57:5:944-947.
21. Kocher, H.C. (1972), "Yoga practices as variable in Neuroticism, Anxiety and Hostility," Yoga Mimamsa, Vol. XV, No. 2, 37-46.
22. Kocher, H.C. (1976), "Anxiety, General Hostility and its Direction as result of yogic practices, Yoga Mimamsa, Vol. XVII, No. 4, 73-82.
23. Kocher, H.C. and Pratap, V. (1971), "Neurotic trend and yogic practices," Yoga Mimamsa, Vol. XIV, No. 1 & 2.
24. Kocher, H.C. and Pratap, V. (1972), "Anxiety level and yogic practice," Yoga Mimamsa, Vol. XV, No. 1, 11-15.
25. Levey and Levey, M. (1987), "The fine arts of relaxation, concentration and meditation," Wisdom Publications, Boston.

26. Mall, N.N., Chaudhary, G.S. and Giri, C. (1976), "Effects of relaxo-concentration training on two psychomotor tasks after submaximal exercise," Paper presented at the VI National Conference of Sports Medicine at Amarawati (Maharashtra).

27. Miller, D.K. and Allen. T.E. (1986), "Fitness: A life time commitment," Edena, MN, Burgess, Publishing.

28. Ministry of education & social welfare (1979), "Draft-National sports Policy prepared by: The All India Council of sports published by Govt. Of India.

29. Pratap, V. (1968), "Steadiness in normals before and after yogic practice–An exploratory study," Yoga Mimamsa, Vol. No. XI; 2; 1-13.

30. Rasch, C.J. (1958), "The functional capacities of a Yoga." Jour. of the American Osteopathic Assoc. 58; 520-523.

31. Rathbone, J.L. (1959), "Corrective physical education," Philadelphia: W.B. Saunders.

32. Rathbone, J.L. (1969), "Relaxation." Lea & Febiger, Philadelphia, Romenovaski, W. and Pasek, T. (1969), "Studies on Physiological and psychological evaluation of yoga system exercises," Physical education and sport., Vol. XIII-No. 3, 139-170.

33. Romanovaski, W. and Pasek, T. (1970), "Tentative introduction of relaxation-concentration Gymnastics according to yoga system as supplementary exercises in physical education of students," Scientific Conf. Medic. faculty, Poznan, 4:24-25.

34. Saraswati, Satyananda, Swami (1994), "Swara-Yoga," Bihar Yoga Vidyalaya, Munger (Bihar).

35. Swami Kuvalyananda, and Vinekar, S.L. (1963), "Yogic therapy–Its basic principles and methods," Central Health Education Bureau, Directorate General of Services, Ministry of Health, Govt. of India, New Delhi.

36. Wallace, R.K. (1970), "Physiological effects of transcendental meditation," Students International Meditation Society, Los Angeles, California.

37. Wallace, R.K. and Benson, H. (1972), "The physiology of meditation, Scientific American, Vol. 226, No. 2.

38. Wenger, M.A. and Bagehi, B.K. (1961), "Studies of autonomic functions in practitioners of yoga in India," Behavioural science, 6:312-323.

39. Vidyalankar, J.D. (Translator) (1944), "Charak Samhita," Vol. I, Motilal Banarasidas, Varanasi (U.P.)

Comparative Study of Effects of Yogic and Non-Yogic Exercises on Selected Physiological Variables of Kabaddi Players

A.N. Khodarkar

Introduction

'Kabaddi' is a traditional popular game of India. It is an unique 'Team Game' in the wold, in which a single individual called 'raider', attacks the opponents team of seven members called 'anti-raiders' in their (opponent's) court. Entry of the raider in opponent's court starts with cant and continues his attack (raiding) upto the limit of his cant.

Cant is repeated in clear sound of approved word 'Kabaddi' within the course of a single expiration. It is prerequisite of the game involving physiological factor which influences the raider's duration. Other skills of the game are greatly influenced by the duration of the cant. The raider who has an ability to continue his cant for longer duration can have better and more opportunities to exhibit his raiding skills. A short duration of the cant puts limit to the raider's attack.

In view of the important role of cant in the game of Kabaddi, it is desirable to find some effective measures to imporve canting ability and endurance of the Kabaddi players.

Present system of training the Kabaddi players includes orthodox and modern sets of exercises. Use of Yogic Exercises in the training schedules of Kabaddi players is rarely found. Canting ability is supposed to be based upon respiratory efficiency and Yogic Practices are known for their contribution to respiratory efficiency. Therefore, to find out the effective measure and compare the effectiveness of Yogic and non-Yogic exercises on physiological variables like Breath holding, Vital Capacity of the Kabaddi players, this experiment was undertaken.

Review of the Literature

The review of the literature pertaining to this topic is to find out the work of Dr. Gharote scientifically investigated on cant. Only a few studies by some researchers and mostly these are related to Yoga and Fitness. Very few studies throw light on the cant ability in the game of Kabaddi. Gharote (5) observed that the training in Yogic Exercises for a period of three weeks definitely improves the general fitness of the male individuals Ganguly *et al.* (6) found that Yogic Training programme improved cardio-vascular efficiency.

In a comparable study between Yogic and non-Yogic exercises Udupa *et al.* (7) found that the vital capacity and vital index along with the body weight and blood pressure increase through both the types of exercises.

Methodology

The study was conducted on 75 male Kabaddi players of age group 18—25 years of local Physical Education Training College.

Their height, weight and birth date were recorded.

After that, all the players were tested through the following tests:

(1) Endurance* (cardio-respiratory)—by Harvard Step Test.

(2) Vital Capacity**—Tested by Spirometer.

* Endurance—is the result of physiological capacity of the individual to sustain movement over a period of time.

** Vital Capacity—is the volume of air that can be expelled by the most forcible exhalation after the deepest inhalation.

(3) Breath Holding Time:

(a) Internal
(b) External
Measured by Stop Watch.

Then these subjects were divided into three groups equally that is Experimental Group 'A' (Yogic Exercise); Group 'B' (non-Yogic Exercise) and Control Group 'C'.

The Yogic Training Programme was given to the Experimental Group 'A' for six weeks for 30 minutes daily except on Sunday. The non-Yogic exercises were given to the 'B' Group for six weeks for 30 minutes daily except on Sunday.

All the groups were being involved in the common physical Education Programme of the College in addition to the Experimental Exercises regularly.

Training Programme

(A) Yogic Training Programme was consisted of the following exercises:

(1) Sarvangasana

(2) Matsyasana

(3) Halasana

(4) Bhujangasana

(5) Salabhasana

(6) Paschimatanasana

(7) Ardh-Matsyendrasana

(8) Dhanurasana

(9) Yoga Mudra

(10) Chakrasana

(11) Mayurasana

(12) Savasana

(13) Uddiyana

(14) Kapalbhati

(15) Ujjai

(B) Non-Yogic Programme was consisted of the following exercises:

(1) Deep Breathing Exercises

(2) Jogging and Spot Running.

(3) Skipping

(4) Dandas

(C) Control Group was not involved in any exercises except their routine programme.

Post Training Tests

After six weeks training programme again all these groups were tested with the same procedure as adopted during the initial tests. Results of the tests were recorded and then the statistical analysis of the data was made to derive conclusion.

Analysis of Data

Following formula was used to calculate the 't' Value to test the difference of means in the performance of the two groups.

Findings

For each of the chosen variables the results pertaining to significant difference, if any, between pre-test and post-test means of the three groups, which are assessed by employing 't' test and analysis of variance has been given below:

Table 1

Significant Differences Between the Pre-Test and Past Test Means of Selected Phisiological Variables of Control Group

Test Item	*Mean value Pre-test*	*Mean value of Post-test*	*'t' value*
Internal Breath Holding	54.34	55.27	1.77
External Breath Holding	33.11	38.37	1.30
Vital Capacity	3364.92	3413.08	2.05
Harvard Step Test Index	84.22	84.89	1.94

Table 2

Significant Differences Between the Pre-Test and Post Test Means of Selected Physiological Variables of Yogic Group

Test Item	*Mean value Pre-test*	*Mean value of Post-test*	*'t' value*
Internal Breath Holding	53.34	65.72	2.45*
External Breath Holding	34.11	42.14	2.84*
Vital Capacity	3684.76	4119.	2.22*
Harvard Step Test	83.67	93.81	3.10*

* Significant at .05 level of confidence.

Table 3

Significant Differences Between the Pre-Test and Post-Test Means of Selected Physiological Variances of Non-Yogic Group

Test Item	*Mean value Pre-test*	*Mean value of Post-test*	*'t' value*
Internal Breath Holding	46.9	57.81	8.33*
External Breath Holding	32.46	39.22	6.66*
Vital Capacity	3293.56	3589.76	11.35*
Harvard Step Test	81.09	83.36	11.35*

* Significant at .05 level of confidence.

The mean differences in the pre-test and post-test in group 'A', group 'B' and group 'C' were analysed by applying 't' test for statistical significance. It is evident from Table 2 & 3 that the groups improved their performance after 6 weeks training. The 't' ratios obtained were found significant at .05 level as it was more than 20.6. There were no significant difference in group 'C'.

Since the experimental groups showed significant increase in performance of selected variables the data were further subjected to analysis of variance to find if there were any significant differences among the groups. The Analysis of variance is shown in Table 4.

Table 4

Analysis of Variance of the Mean Differences in Selected Physiological Variables

Variables:	*Source of Variance:*	*d f:*	*sum of: mean*	*sum of: square*	*'F' value*
Internal Breath Holding	Among groups	2	1490.07	745.04	3.08
	Within groups	72	17441.85	242.25	
External Breath Holding	Among groups	2	247.09	123.55	0.87
	Within groups	72	10195.02	141.59	
Vital Capacity	Among groups	2	156897./	78448.5	7.42*
	Within groups	72	760802./	10566.69	
Harward Step Test	Among groups	2	1858.84	929.42	16.05*
	Within groups	72	4167.36	57.83	

* Significant at .05 level of confidence (2.72) 3.13.

Table 4 revealed that there are significant differences in vital capacity and Harward step test were obtained 'F' ratio are 7.42 and 16.05 which are much higher value than the value 3.13 required for 'F' ratio to the significant at 9.05 level with (2.72) degree of freedom.

As the 'F' ratios are found significant in the case of vital capacity and Hardward step test, the scheffe's post-hoc test was applied to test the significance of differences which are presented in following Tables 5 & 6.

Table 5

Paired Adjusted Final Means and Differences Between Means for Three Groups in Vital Capacity

Yogic	*Non-Yogic*	*Control*	*M.D.*
4115.08	3589.76		525.32*
4115.08		3453.09	661.39*
	3589.76	3453.09	136.67*

*Significant at .05 level. The critical difference at .05 level is 72.68.

Table 6

Paired Adjusted Final Means and Differences Between Means for Three Groups in H.S. Test

Yogic	*Non-Yogic*	*Control*	*M.D.*
95.01	83.96		11.05*
95.01		83.72	11.29*
	83.96	83.72	.24

* Significant at .05 level of confidence. The C.D. at .05 level is 5.38.

Discussion

We found that in almost all the tests, experimental groups have recorded better performance than the Control group. As well as it is also found that performance of the experimental group 'A' is more better than the performance of the group 'B'.

From the present study, it is concluded that Yogic exercises have better effect than the non-Yogic exercises. It is also concluded that Yogic exercises are better to improve the physiological variables than non-Yogic exercises.

Recommendation

It is suggested that Yogic training programme be included in the training schedule of the Kabaddi players along with the non-Yogic exercises for getting better results.

References

1. Bucher, C.A., *Foundation of Physical Education,* Saint Louis: C.V. Mosby Company, 1972.
2. Mathews, D.K., Measurement in Physical Education, Saint Louis,
3. Falls, H.B., Exercise Physiology, New York: Academic Press, 1968.
4. Gharote, M.L., *Cant in Kabaddi*—A Study, SNIPES Journal Vol. 4, No. 3 (July 81).
5. Gharote, M.L., Effect of Yogic Training on Physical Fitness, Y.M. Vol. XV, Jan., 1973; pp. 31-35.
6. Ganguly, S.K. and Gharote, M.L., Cardio Vascular efficiency before and after Yogic Training, Y.M. Vol. XVII (April, 1974), pp. 89-97.

7. Udupa, K.N., Singh, R.H., and Settiwar, R.M., A Comparative Study on the Effect of Some Individual Yogic Practices in Normal Persons, I.J. Med., Res., 63,8, pp. 1066-1071, August, 1975.

8. Gharote, M.L., *Guidelines for Yogic Practices,* Medha Publication, Lonavla 1982.

9. Gopal, K.S., Bhatnagar, C.P., Subramanian, N. and Nishith, S.D., Effect of Yogasanas & Pranayama on Blood Pressure, Pulse Rate & Some Respiratory Functions, Indian Journal of Physiological Pharmacology, 17, pp. 273-276, 1973.

10. Swami Kuvalayananda, Asana, Kaivalyadhama, Lonavla.

Relaxation

Vimla Vagrecha

Modern age is the era of anxiety, tension, and fatigue. Everybody is in a rush. He has not time to think at leisure and he has to do so many things to survive. Everything is time bound and man is running after them to get ahead. This makes him tired physically and tense mentally. In order to get rid of physical fatigue and mental tension, man has devised certain means. He goes to parties, drink there and see movies. But here also instead of getting relaxation he comes with more tension and fatigue. Purchased relaxation won't give him relief. It increases his trouble. Then what? If one is tired, fatigued but continue to work, it is said that the damage will be three-fold—physical, mental and emotional. That is the reason, relaxation is very much advocated. Ancient Yogis realizing that mind and body required rest, advocated relaxation for healthy living.

Napoleon Bonaparte was master in the art of relaxation. In the battle field, during war, he used to sleep and rest completely for 5 minutes on the horse back and then used to fight again with renewed energy.

Mahatma Gandhi was another person in the recent past who was knowing this art very well. Before any important meeting, he used to relax completely for 5 to 10 minutes.

It is important to realize that it is the mind which plays havoc. Till mind is not given rest we can't relax, that is the reason that picnic, parties and movies or any other sort of purchased relaxation give more tiredness and tension as in these activities mind is overtaxed instead of getting rest.

Modern Yoga is based on relaxation and rhythm. All Yogic exercises, Asanas and pranayams are rhythmic and give relaxation. However, there are certain specific Asans which are meant completely for relaxation. These are very much beneficial for heart action, fall in blood pressure and pulse rate, evenness of respiratory activities and lowers the circulation of blood in the brain and thus cause sedative effect. These practices which are entirely or exclusively meant for relaxation are called *Psycho-somatic* or *neuro-mascular* practices.

Relaxation really means rest after efforts, more truly, conscious rest after conscious efforts and it does not mean lying in a lazy manner or doing nothing. It means a complete resignation of the body to the laws of gravity, the mind to nature, and the whole energy transferred to a deep dynamic breathing. The complete relaxation of the voluntary muscles at once transfers the energy to the involuntary parts, so in the strict sense, there is not relaxation, but bringing an equilibrium between voluntary actions and involuntary reactions for the renewal of strength. Relaxation gives the maximum amount of renewed strength in the minimum amount of time. Even more than sleep, successful relaxation is the vital principle of rest, which quickly regalvanizes the nerves centres and reinvigorates the whole body.

Whenever physical or mental fatigue or strain is experienced, or the mind is agitated, the practice of certain postures are recommended. These are as follows—

(i) **Savasan** or the corpse-pose : Lying sapine, face towards the sky, arms at sides with the legs passively extended to their full length. It can by *(i)* partial *(ii)* total.

(ii) **Dradhasana** or the firm pose: It is practised by lying on the right side of the body in a state of relaxation with the right arm under the head as a pillow.

(iiii) **Makarasana** or the crocodile pose: It consists in lying prostrate with the chest, the abdoment and the front

of the body in close contact with the floor—the legs at full length and apart, the arms folded and the head resting thereon.

(iv) **Nispand Bhav**: While sitting and relaxed get into the listening mood and let the sound come to you. You need not reach to sound.

It is the state of mind which disturbs us. We can not control totally outside world, but we can inculcate the habit in ourselves to have passivity of mind so the outside factors won't disturb us.

Many things happen in the family and we react towards it, which creates unhappiness and quarrels. In order not to react passivity of mind is required.

One proverbial story is very useful in this regard.Once a man was going in a forest where he met with a monkey. The monkey told him that he will do every thing for him, but the moment there will be nothing to do for him, he will eat the master. The man was very happy. For days together man ordered him to do several work and kept him busy but after all there was an end of the work. Man got worried that now the monkey will eat him. So ultimately man asked the monkey to bring a ladder and keep on climbing up and getting down till further orders.

The mind is just like a monkey. Mind has a vicious hold and circle on the body. Even in the sleep mind won't loose the hold of body. Mind cannot be kept blank but to loosen the hold of mind upon body we have to keep mind busy in something—listening—and thus loosen the hold of the mind on the body.

In modern time, there is so much noise pollution that if we are bombarded with all these probably we will be mad. Some screening is necessary. Physiological and mental homiostasis does it automatically. Still we are subjected to too many things. Through practice of Nispand Bhav we can inculcate the habit to listen only desired things.

Apart from the above specific Asans other Yogic exercises also have a relaxing effect in comparison to non-Yoga exercises as stated below.

Yoga

1. Yoga physical exercises are *static* one. It won't require off-repeated contractions and relaxations of the muscles. Hence, economizing the energy and all round development.
2. Yoga physical exercise are *organismic.* They give exercise to the internal as well as external organs equally. The more emphasis is upon the exercises of internal organs which are often remain neglected during day-to day physical movements.
3. **Anabotic:** Yoga physical exercise conserve the biological energy, it restores it rather than to spend it.
4. Yoga physical exercise give calmness and relaxation. It soothens the mind and body both and have *sadative* effect.
5. **Subjective:** The good effects of Yoga exercises are felt and experienced pleasantly.
6. **Extramundane:** It leads to travel withing self, refinement of consciousness and detachment to worldly affairs.

Non-Yoga

1. Non-Yoga physical exercises are *repetative* in nature. There is continuous contractions and relaxation of certain muscles of the body, which give rise to un-equal growth of the body muscles and consume more energy in exercises.
2. Non-Yoga pysical exercises gives exercise to external muscles only and internal organs, so vital for maintenance of total health remain un-touched.
3. **Katabolic:** Great amount of bio-energy get exhausted in non-Yoga physical exercises, it spends more energy than to restore.
4. Non-Yoga physical exercises, by putting more blood circulation in the brain and in certain body part make the organism in an *agitative* state.
5. **Objective:** The effect of N.Y.P.E. are more visible, lead to competitiveness.

6. **Mundane:** leads to animality, worldly attachment and more possessiveness.

Therefore, specific and non-specific Yogic exercises and attitude are very much beneficial for relaxation which is absolutely essential in modern era of stress and strain to survive and to function effectively.

Bibliography

Shri Yogendra (1980). Yoga Asanas Simplified. Bombay: The Yoga Institute.

A New Light on Haṭhapradīpikā

M.L. Gharota

Introduction

Haṭhapradīpikā is an important treatise on Haṭhayoga written by Svātmārāma and has commanded a great influence not only on the practical students of yoga but also has become a source of inspiration for many later writers on Haṭhayoga as can be seen from the treaties like Yogacintāmaṇi, Haṭharatnāvali, Haṭhasaṅketacandrikā and Haṭhatatta Kaumudī. Several manuscripts are found deposited in the oriental libraries in India and abroad. The first printed edition of Haṭhapradīpikā was brought out by Tukārāma Tātyā of Bombay in 1893. Several Indian and foreign editions are more or less the reproduction of similar text with the exception of the critical edition brought out by the Kaivalyadhāma S.M.Y.M. Samiti, Lonavla in 1970. The efforts made for this critical edition are noteworthy because 101 manuscripts preserved in different libraries were consulted for preparing this edition. This critical edition contains 5 chapters, the last one describing the therapeutical remedies of the complaints of the yogic practitioners as a result of faulty yogic practices. This last chapter is not found in any of the printed edition of the Haṭhapradīpikā.

The Special Features of the Fifth Chapter

The fifth chapter in Kaivalyadhāma critical edition of Haṭhapradīpikā is devoted to the treatment of disorders caused by the erroneous practice of yoga. The type of disorders mentioned therein are: chest pain, pain in the sides, backache, headache, asthma, hiccup, skin disease, partial blindness, tremors, blood infection etc. The terminology of the diseases as well as their etiology is Āyurvedic. These disease are attributed to the faulty coursing of the Vāyu in the upward direction and blocking of the energy. The suggested treatment in general is to concentrate on the part where the trouble exists. This is in the form of visualization technique. The other methods of treatment suggested are:

(1) Practice of Pūraka and Recaka.

(2) Taking a lubricating diet.

(3) Practising breath-holding 2-3 times after taking the food.

(4) Warm food prepared in milk with ghee and practising Vāruṇī dhāraṇā.

(5) Liquid food with ghee.

(6) Increasing the intensity of the yogic practice.

(7) Massage with oil and bath with hot water.

It has also been suggested that an adequate help of medicine be taken wherever necessary along with yogic treatment.

Although this fifth chapter deals with yogic treatment, it is doubtful whether this chapter originally forms a part of the Haṭhapradīpikā. It deals with the Nādānusandhāna and Rājayoga topics. However, it is very informative.

The Scope of Haṭhapradīpikā

It is to be noted that different manuscripts of Haṭhapradīpikā vary in their contents. Some manuscripts contain a few verses which are not found in other manuscripts. What could be the source of the variance in these verses? Could there be other copies of the text of Haṭhapradīpikā different from the published one?

The purpose of this presentation is to throw light on this issue.

How many chapters are contained in the Haṭhapradīpikā? In all the published texts of Haṭhapradīpikā and in many

Table 1

Number of Chapters and Verses in Different Texts of Haṭhapradīpikā

	Text	*Number of Chapters*	*Number of Verses*	*Special Features*
1.	Adyār Library and Research Center Text (published)	4	389	
2.	Kaivalyadhāma Text (published)	5	409	Description of yogic treatment
3.	India Office Library London (manuscript)	4	401	
4.	Oxford University Library (manuscript)	4	331	
5.	Mahārājā Mānsingh Library, Jodhpur (manuscript)	10	643	Pratyāhāra, Rājayoga, Kālajñāna, Videhamukti
6.	Rājasthān Oriental Research Institute Jodhpur (manuscript)	6	1553	Characteristics of Guru-śiṣya, Description of more than 100 āsanas, Rules of Diet, Description of Kanda-Nāḍi-Kuṇḍalinī, unlucky omens of death and means of control.

unpublished manuscripts we get four chapters. But there are other texts available which give different number of chapters and their verses also vary in number.

Table 1 gives the number of chapters and verses in different texts.

Kavikāvyakālakalpanā mentions 500 verses of Haṭhapradīpikā.

From Table 1 it will be clear that the contents of Haṭhapradīpikā are variously distributed in 4, 5, 6 or 10 chapters and that the verses in different texts greatly vary. Although Mahārājā Mānsingh Library Ms. contains largest number of chapters, the number of verses, however, are lesser than the Rājasthān Oriental Research Library manuscript which has 1553 verses distributed in 6 chapters and is the largest manuscript available. It is desirable that first we get aquainted with the contents of this manuscript.

Description of the R.O.R.I. Jodhpur Manuscript

This manuscript is numbered 6756, size 17 cm x 9 cm, pages 171, lines 7-9 and letters 20-23.

The colophon reads:

"Iti śri sahajanāth śiṣyeṇa śri Svātmārāmayogīndreṇa viracitāyāṃ Haṭhapradīpikāyāṃ siddhāntamuktāvalyāṃ ṣaṣṭhopadeśaḥ iti/śrirastu/Śrimanmahārājādhirāja śri Jayasiṃhadevajikasyājñayā likhitamidam Tulārāmeṇa saṃvat 1765 varṣe caitre māse kṛṣṇa pakṣe 10 śrīrāmo jayati/sri Gaṇapataye namaḥ/

There are some faults of the scribe but the text is generally correct. The distribution of the verses and contents in each chapter as compared with the Kaivalyadhāma printed edition is shown in Table 2.

The topics not found discussed in the printed edition of Haṭhapradīpikā but available in the Jodhpur manuscript are presented in Table 3. It is to be noted that the contents of the fifth chapter in Kaiva lyadhāma printed edition related to the therapeutical application are conspicuously absent in the Jodhpur manuscript.

Table 2

Number of Verses in Each Chapter of Haṭhapradīpikā

Haṭhapradīpikā Jodhpur Ms.			*Haṭhapradīpikā Kaivalyadhāma Printed Edition*		
Chp. No.	*No. Verses*	*Contents*	*Chp. No.*	*No. Verses*	*Contents*
I	177	Hathayoga–Rājayoga relationship, need of Haṭhayoga, List of adepts practicing Hathayoga, Importance of practice according to the Shashtra and as directed by the Guru, Eulogy and characteristics of Sadguru, Characteristics of a bad disciple, Need of behaviour as prescribed by Dharma.	I	67	Haṭhayoga–Rājayoga relationship, Characteristics of Yogic hut, Description of Āsanas, Haṭhayoga curriculum and Yogic diet.
II	136	Characteristics of suitable region and Yogic hut for the practice, Yogasiddhi and asiddhi lakshanas, Yama-Niyama, Curriculum of Hathayoga, Description of 97 Asanas, Rules of diet and contraindicated food.	II	78	Prāṇāyāma–its utility and description of 8 varieties, Description and effects of six purificatory processes, Description and eulogy of Kevala Kumbhaka and symptoms of the success in Haṭhayogic practices.
III	200	Importance and eulogy of Prāṇāyāma.	III	126	Description and effects of 10 mudrās for the awakening of Kuṇḍalini.
IV	138	Efficacy of Ṣatkarmas and their technique description of the eight varieties of Kumbhaka, purpose of Prāṇāyāma.	IV	114	Rājayoga or Samādhi by conducting Prāṇa through Suṣumnā by resorting to various techniques but emphasing on Nādānusandhāna, contribution of Śāmbhavi and Khecari and various stages of attaining progress in laya.

V	543	Description of Kanda, three Naḍis and Kuṇḍalini, discussion on 10 mudrās with elaborate description of Khecari.	V	24	Treatment of the disorders due to erroneous yogic practices. This topic is found only in 2 manuscripts.
VI	364	Description of various techniques of Dhyāna leading to Samādhi. Emphasis on Nādānusandhāna, Advaitayoga. Four stages of absorption of Mind, Internal and external symptoms and unlucky omen indicating time of death, control of death.			
Total1553				409	

Excess Verses 1144

In Table 4 are shown number of additional verses devoted to different topics in the Jodhpur manuscript.

Salient Points

As has been shown the special feature of the Jodhpur manuscript is that it contains not only largest number of verses but also number of topics which are missing in the printed edition. It is worth recording the new information available in this manuscript.

(i) Greatest number of Asanas not described in any traditional text is found in this manuscript. A list of Asanas described is presented in Table 5. Names of some of the Asanas are quite unfamiliar and are not known.

(ii) Under the description of Prāṇāyāma a mention is made of Candrabheda Kumbhaka and Bhujaṅgama Kumbhaka, the latter being the synonym for Sītkāra Kumbhaka which is advocated to be practised any time. This kind of advice is given for the practice of Ujjāyī in the printed edition.

(iii) The text is full of useful quotations and advice. It emphasises on the fact that practice of Āsanas is only a step on the path of Yoga. It says–"A person who only practises Āsanas and not even Prāṇāyāma, throughout the life he goes astray from Yoga and his life becomes useless."

The term "Āsana" has also been used for the 'seat' of which varied description is found.

(iv) As compared to the printed edition the end in this manuscript seems to be more appropriate.

There is also another copy of this text deposited in the R.O.R.I., Jaipur vide No. 3471. But it could not be compared with the Jodhpur text.

On the Commentaries of the Haṭhapradīpikā

The following commentaries on Haṭhapradīpikā have been mentioned in literature:

(1) Haṭhayogapradīpikā ṭīkā Rāmānandatīrtha.

(2) Haṭhapradīpikā Ṭippaṇa by Umāpti.

(3) Haṭhapradīpikā commentary by Mahādeva.
(4) Haṭhapradīpikā commentary (in Hindi) by Vrajabhūṣaṇa.
(5) Haṭhapradīpikāvṛtti (in Marāṭhi) by Bhojātmaja.
(6) Haṭhapradīpikāvyākhyā Jyotsnā by Brahmānanda.

Out of these 1, 2, 3 and 4 are not available. The well-known commentary on the Haṭhapradīpikā is Jyotsnā by Brahmānanda which is published by the Theosophical Publishing House, Adyār, Madras. Along with the commentary of Brahmānanda the other commentaries also seem to comment on the text which is available in the printed form. For Brahmānanda the text of Jodhpur manuscript was not known although it existed before the time of Brahmānanda. Therefore we do not find any commentary on the largest text of Jodhpur manuscript. Brahmānanda belongs to 19th century while the Jodhpur text belongs to 18th century.

Recently we have come across another commentary in Sanskrit on Haṭhapradīpikā written by Bālakṛṣṇa which is deposited in the Mahārājā Mānsingh Library, Jodhpur vide No. 2228. It is named as "Yogaprakāśikā" and is a commentary on the text of Haṭhapradīpikā having 10 chapters, also deposited in the same library vide No. 2227. The special feature of this text of Haṭhapradīpikā is the discussion on the topics of Pratyāhāra, Rājayoga, Kālajñāna and Videhamukti.

On the basis of the new information available about the text of Haṭhapradīpikā a question arises as to which text should be considered as original. For a long time the Adyār edition of Haṭhapradīpikā containing 4 chapters has been recognised as the original text until the critical edition of Haṭhapradīpikā from Kaivalyadhāma appeared in 1970 which has a fifth chapter in addition. However, after getting the two manuscripts of Haṭhapradīpikā from Jodhpur, reconsideration about the original text has become necessary.

In the preface about the critical edition of Haṭhapradīpikā from Kaivalyadhāma, the editors wrote–

"In Gorakṣasiddhānta-saṅgraha (p. 38) there is a reference to Haṭhapradīpikā having as many as ten chapters. But we have not yet come across any manuscript of this text covering more than five chapters. There is a crying need for further research aimed at finding a complete or differently arranged but exhaustive version of this important text."

With the new information available it is possible to reconstruct the original exhaustive version of the Haṭhapradīpikā.

One of the problems that arises out of the colophon of Jodhpur manuscript is the relation of Siddhānta-muktāvali with Haṭhapradīpikā. Although we do not get the mention of the Siddhāntamuktāvali in the colophon of the printed text, there are at least ten manuscripts which have the mention of Siddhāntamuktāvali along with Haṭhapradīpikā. What has Haṭhapradīpikā to do with Siddhānta? The word 'Siddhānta' refers to a work to be studied by those who seek self-realisation. (Bṛ. Yāj. Smṛ. XII-35). From this point of view Svātmārāma considers Haṭhapradīpikā as a Siddhānta grantha of Haṭhayoga. He also mentions in the end of the text as follows:

> "Haṭhapradīpikāṃ śrutvā siddhānta granthamuttamam/
> tyaktvā bhrāntimaśāstrāṇi satāṃ sadyaḥ parāṃ gatiḥ//"

In order to emphasize that this treatise on Haṭhayoga is a Siddhāntagrantha, he seems to mention this fact in the colophon of each chapter.

Conclusion

In the light of the above discussion it may be suggested that the Jodhpur manuscript represents original text of Haṭhapradīpikā. It was also called Siddhāntamuktāvali. In the later recessions much of the contents of the text was left out and the text was abridged. We have no means to acertain whether Svātmārāma himself was responsible for this abridgement or someone else. The mention of Siddhāntamuktāvali along with Haṭhapradīpikā in the colophon continued for sometime and later the name of Siddhāntamuktāvali was dropped out from the colophon. Along with the abridgement of the text, the process of reorganisation of the contents and dividing them into suitable chapters from 4 to 10 continued. Thus, the text of Haṭhapradīpikā seems to have passed through at least 3 or 4 stages. But for the elaborate description and contents of the text we should turn our attention to Jodhpur manuscript. There is a need of reconstructing the text of Haṭhapradīpikā using the Jodhpur manuscript as vulgate text.

"योग द्वारा सर्वांगीण विकास"

विपुल भट्ट

पहला सुख निरोगी काया यह कहा गया है। पाश्चात्य देशों में भी "Health is Wealth" कहकर स्वस्थ शरीर की महिमा गायी गई है। कौन नहीं चाहता संसार के सभी सुखों का वह भोग करे, किन्तु वे ही ऐसा कर पाते हैं जिनके पास स्वस्थ शरीर, शान्त मन, आत्मविश्वास, व चरित्र बल है। दुनियाँ में किसी के पास अपार बल है तो मन अशान्त है। किसी के पास अपार धन राशि है पर स्वस्थता नहीं । किसी के पास चिन्ता है, संतान-हीनता, आत्मग्लानि और न जाने कितने ही ऐसे क्लेश हैं जिसके कारण हर कोई दुखी है। किन्तु जो अन्दर व बाहर से सुखी हैं अर्थात् जिसे निरोग शरीर व आत्म शान्ति प्राप्त है, उसे अन्य किसी वस्तुओं में सुख नहीं खोजना पड़ता। तो इसी अंतरिम एवं बाह्य स्वस्थता को कायम रखने हेतु, किये जाने वाले अभ्यास को योग की संज्ञा दी गई है।

योग में न ही किसी मैदान की, आडंबर की, उपकरणों की, धन की, सहयोगियों की अर्थात् किसी की भी आवश्यकता नहीं होती। परन्तु खेल या अन्य व्यायाम में मैदान की, पैसा की, सहयोगियों की या उपकरणों की आवश्यकता होती है। हां जो मजदूरी करते हैं, जैसे बढ़ई या लुहारी कार्य, हाथ ठेला चलाना आदि कार्य नियमित रूप से करते हैं, वे हमारे इसी अभ्यास के क्रम में आते हैं। परन्तु वे शान्त चित्त हों ही यह जरूरी नहीं। योग हेतु हमें थोड़ी सी जगह, 20 मिनट का समय (चाहे प्रातःकाल या सांध्य का कोई भी समय) एवं स्थिर व शान्त मन यही कुल चाहिये। हड़बड़ी, जल्दबाजी, दिखावा, चिन्तायुक्त, मस्तिष्क रोगी तो योग हेतु कदापि नहीं। स्वयं को ऊपर उठाने, समाज में योग्य व्यक्ति कहलाने, चरित्र के बल संयम व अभ्यास नियमन से राष्ट्र को गौरान्वित करने वाला व्यक्ति का निर्माण करना ही योग का अंतिम लक्ष्य है।

भारत शासन एवं कई राज्यों ने इसलिये योग को, शिक्षा नीति के अंतर्गत, योग विज्ञान निरूपित कर प्रशिक्षण केन्द्रों, कालेजों व स्कूलों में एक विषय मान पठन-पाठन हेतु अनिवार्य विषय माना है। इससे योग की महत्ता अपने आप समझ में आती है। योग केवल शरीर को निरोगी ही नहीं रखता, वरन् योग करने वाले को प्राय: हृदय रोग जैसा रोग कभी नहीं हो सकता, जो आज के युग में अभिशाप का रूप ले चुका है। योग के चमत्कारी गुणों में मन, मस्तिष्क, फेफड़े, हृदय, अमाशय, यकृत, रक्त ग्रन्थियां, गुर्दे, रक्त संचालन, मल-मूत्र विसर्जन व चरित्र को विशेष बल मिलता है, जिससे मनुष्य शान्त, सुन्दर, निरोग, दीर्घायु, विवेकशील, स्मरणशक्ति वाला एक आत्मविश्वासी व्यक्तित्व का धनी बन जाता है।

योग अभ्यास दस वर्ष की आयु से अंतिम समय तक किया जा सकता है। किन्तु शर्त यही है कि आप किसी गंभीर व्याधि से ग्रसित न हों। प्राकृतिक नियमों की अवहेलना करने से शरीर रोग ग्रस्त होता है। अत: योग नियमित, अनुशासित, एकाग्रचित्त एवं खाली पेट ही करना अत्यन्त आवश्यक है। योग के माध्यम से जहां एक ओर कब्ज, एसीडिटी, जुखाम, बुखार, अतिसार, गठिया-वात, मधुमेह, धातरोग आदि व्याधियों का उपचार कर छुटकारा पा सकते हैं। वहीं सुचारु रूप से रक्त संचार, श्वसन, रस ग्रन्थियों की सक्रियता, मस्तिरूक का बौद्धिक विकास, स्मरण शक्ति, मन में शान्ति, आत्मविश्वास सहज ही प्राप्त किया जा सकता है वहीं मोह, ईर्ष्या, क्रोध आदि से दूर रहकर अपने को एक उत्साही, साहसी, स्वाभिमानी, निरोग, चरित्रवान व्यक्ति भी बनाया जा सकता है।

शरीर संपदा उत्कर्षता की अवस्था है, मनुष्य शरीर, संसार का सबसे बड़ा आश्चर्य है। शरीर को सभी धर्म, जाति, अमीर-गरीब एक सा ही धारण करते हैं अत: योग उपर्युक्त में से किसी को भी बाधा नहीं मानता। वह सभी वर्गों स्त्री-पुरुष, जवान-बूढ़े, प्रौढ़ या बच्चों द्वारा संपादित किया जा सकता है। हाँ, यह जरूरी है कि यह किसी अच्छे पथ-प्रदर्शक के सानिध्य में शुरू करना चाहिये व क्रमश: स्वयं को ही पथ-प्रदर्शक बनाने का प्रयास होना चाहिये, खाने के बाद योग को कदापि न करें। रोगी होने पर, क्रोध या अशान्त होने पर भी योग न करें। बल्कि कुछ देर रुककर स्थिर होने पर यह किया जा सकता है। योग में खान-पान, सदाचार, चरित्र व नैतिकता पर भी विशेष ध्यान दिया गया है। कहा गया है ''जैसा खाओ अन्न वैसा हो मन।'' योग विशेष रूप से अपने शरीर को अन्दर बाहर से स्वच्छ, संतुलित, क्रियाशील, आत्मविश्वासी बनाने का नाम है। आज संसार इस योग विषय के पीछे दीवाना है, और वह दिन दूर नहीं जब योग स्वयं एक-चमत्कारिक साधना व रोग मुक्ति का परम उच्च कोटि का साधन

पूरे संसार में माना जायेगा। कितना ही अच्छा हो कि राष्ट्र के हर व्यक्ति के हेतु योग अनिवार्य कर दिया जाये। चीन जैसे राष्ट्र में रेडियो/टेलीविजन द्वारा प्रत्येक व्यक्ति को शारीरिक व्यायाम एक नियत समय पर करना अनिवार्य ही नहीं, न करने वाले को दण्डनीय भी माना गया है। इस प्रक्रिया से पूरे भारत में अच्छे स्वास्थ्य की प्राप्ति का 50 प्रतिशत समाधान अपने आप ही हो जायेगा। अत्याचार, व्यभिचार, कोर्ट कचहरी, मार-पीट, मोह-लोभ, जैसी कितनी ही बुराईयों पर नियन्त्रण स्वयं ही आ जायेगा। प्राचीन काल के गुरुकुल आश्रम हमारे आज के आदर्श बन गये हैं, अच्छे नागरिक व सुन्दर व्यक्तित्त्व जैसा निर्माण कार्य कर सकते हैं। आवश्यकता केवल दृण इच्छा शक्ति की है। जापान जैसा देश राष्ट्र चरित्र निर्माण का संसार में सर्वोच्च उदाहरण है। हम आप अन्य राष्ट्रों का मार्ग दर्शन करने वाले, पूर्व के आर्यावृत की भांति पुनः वैसा ही क्यों नहीं बन सकते यह एक मनन का विषय है।

उपर्युक्त तथ्यों से यह स्पष्ट हो गया है कि योग जीवन की एक ऐसी सतत् क्रिया है जिसके द्वारा हम अपनी जीवन यात्रा सुखद, निरापद, एवं कांतिमय बना सकते हैं। पुराने समय में ऋषि-मुनियों के पास योग साधना के द्वारा शरीर को रोग मुक्त रखने तक ही शिक्षा सीमित नहीं होती थी, बल्कि इस प्रणाली से वे जीव के परलोक सुधार की बात करते थे। तो जिस योग में इतनी शक्ति हो वह इस लोक के अलावा जीव के कल्याण की बात कह सके, वह विद्या कितनी गंभीर, सक्षम एवं विस्मयकारी होगी। इसकी सहज ही कल्पना की जा सकती है। भारत में प्राचीन काल में घेरण्ड द्वारा योग की कई कठिन एवं चमत्कारी शक्तियों के बारे में विस्तार से लिखा जा चुका है। तद्उपरांत भारत में शिवानन्द, क़ुबल्यानंद, विवेकानंद, श्री अरविन्द, महर्षि महेश योगी और न जाने कितने ही ऐसे विद्वान इस विद्या पर अपनी पुस्तकों के माध्यम से प्रकाश डाल चुके हैं।

अभी भी भारत में कहीं ऐसे योग साधक हैं, जो अपनी सतायु उम्र के बावजूद इस क्रिया में लीन हैं एवं दूरस्थ अंचलों में अपना सुखद जीवन यापन कर रहे हैं। योग स्वयं के उत्थान के अलावा परोपकार का भी एक उत्तम साधन है, क्योंकि जो योग करेगा वह किसी का अहित करने की बात कभी नहीं सोचता। अतः सभी इस साधना में लग जायें तो कितनी ऐसी समस्यायें हैं, जो अपने आप हल हो जायें। विवेकानंद ऐसे कर्मयोगी थे, जो अपने जीवन के अंतिम क्षणों तक इस साधना में रत रहे। आज उनके द्वारा दर्शाये गये योग के महत्व को सभी स्वीकारते हैं। अरविंद ने तो अपने जीवन का लक्ष्य योग की पूर्णता हेतु अर्पण कर दिया। कुबल्यानंद एवं शिवानंद के बारे में कौन नहीं जानता वो तो शाश्वत योग के प्रतिरूपी हैं।

विभिन्न योग अभ्यासों द्वारा जैसे आसन, प्राणायाम, यम-नियम आदि आज के युग में अमृत तुल्य साधना है। किन्तु इस देश का दुर्भाग्य कहिये कि हम अपनी इस प्राचीन धरोहर को जीवित रखने के लिये संघर्ष कर रहे हैं, तो ऐसी विषम परिस्थिति में यदि शिक्षा में योग अनिवार्य किया जाये, तो संभव है। हमारी यह प्राचीनतम प्रणाली आज देश के युवाओं को तन-मन एवं आत्म बल प्रदान कर सकती है। वैसे भी आज जब औसत आयु 65 वर्ष है, एवं 45 वर्ष के बाद हर मनुष्य निढाल सा नजर आता है तब यही एक योग की आशा की किरण हमें इस पतन से बचा पाने का उपाय सुझाती है। आज की शिक्षा अनिवार्य रूप से योग शिक्षा के रूप में होनी चाहिये ताकि बचपन से ही बालक-बालिकाओं में स्वयं को एवं परिचितों को सुन्दर जीवन यापन का तरीका बता सकें।

आज हमारे देश में योग को बढ़ावा देने के लिए कई योजनायें बनाई गई हैं, जिनके लागू हो जाने के बार हमारे देश के शैक्षणिक संस्थानों में योग की शिक्षा अनिवार्य रूप से होगी।

Part IV

PHILOSOPHICAL ASPECT OF YOGA

Concept of Personality in Patanjali

Radhavallabh Tripathi

Sanskrit language does not have any word for personality in the modern sense of the term. The word *vyaktitva* has been coined for it in modern Indian languages, which is not a correct usage according to Paninian system of grammar. *Vyakti* does not mean an individual in Sanskrit. In fact individualism and individualistic tendencies do not find a place in our Philosophy, which postulates the theory of infinity. *"Yo vai bhuma tat sukham na alpe sukham asti"*–Bliss lies where there is infinity, bliss does not find place in meagreness–says the Upanisad. Rightly therefore, personality-cult as such did not develop in this tradition.

However, personality is not altogether overruled in this philosophy. Rather there is emphasis on understanding human personality and its immense potential in its right perspective and in totality. Human body is the base for the expression and growth of personality. All systems of Indian philosophy analyse this body, its various organs and functioning. In fact the vedic seers have presented the concept of human personality in all its complicated structure and comprehensiveness. **Atharvaveda** says

> Pundarikam navadvaram tribhir gunebhiravrtam.
> Tasminyad yaksam atanvat tad vai brahmavidi viduh.
>
> *(Atharva. X.8.43)*

Kathopanishad has given a picturesque and metaphorical description of human personality. Accordingly, body is the chariot, the organs are horses, the mind is the reign, wisdom is the charioteer and the soul is the owner of the chariot. If we take out soul out of this metaphor, then the picture that emerges comes very close to the modern concept of human personality. We can also place the complete picture presented by the *upanishad* in contrast to this picture sans-soul. The concept of human personality as visualised in the aupanishadic tradition, places soul over and above all other components.

Modern Psychology differentiates between the brain and the mind. Brain is the machine and the mind is its driven. Here the metaphor of the chariot and the charioteer is recast in a different context, but there is no power supervising both. What appears to be the most animate part of human personality in Western thinking, has been taken up as inanimate in itself in *Samkhya-Yoga* systems. Decartes postulates the theory of a spiritual Soul which is above and beyond mind and thought. Like the theory of *Chichchhayapatti,* he presented the theory of Interactionism, establishing a link between this so-called spiritual soul and the mind and thought power on the other. However, no specific reason or purpose has been defined by Descartes behind this process of interaction. In *Samkhya* and Yoga, *Prakriti* initiates this process of *Chichchhayapatti* or linkage between the pure consciousness and the mind etc. for the pleasure *(bhoga)* and salvation *(moksa)* of the *Purusha* or pure consciousness. *Purusha* is inactive, only because of his supervision, he appears to assuming the activity. **Vijnanabhikshu** has defined this superimposition of activity on the *Purusha* through the example of the iron and magnet. The magnet is not active in itself, but when it comes into the contact with the iron, it empowers the iron. In the same way, the Purusha is not active in itself, but when it comes into the contact with the mind, it infuses its consciousness in the latter.

The relationship between the *Purusha* and the mind has been variously defined by the latter authors who have written *Bhashyas* on Patanjalli's system. **Vyasabhashya** says that the *Purusha* remains isolated from the mind and its thought-process. He just sees. Seeing the mind and its process defines his relationship with them. The author of **Yogavartika** however visualises the relationship as *bimba-pratibimba-bhve, i.e.* the *Purusha* is the original and the mind is its reflection.

As a result of this *bimba-pratibimbabhava* a proximity is established between *Purusha* and *Prakriti* so that *Purusha* begins to feel himself effected by the experiences of happiness or sorrow through which the sense-organs undergo, and he takes himself to have become happy, unhappy or subjected by worldly pleasures or pains. *(Vyasabhashya on Patanjalayogasutra 1,4;* Varanasi, 1981, p.3).

The author of *Yogavartika* has given a novel interpretation to this relationship of *bimba-pratibimbabhava* between *purusha* and *prakriti.* He says that this relationship is reciprocal. There is reflection of conscious-being in vrtti, and then this reflection produces counter image in conscious being. In this way, there is an unending chain of reflections and counter reflections, where the *purusha* and *vrtti* stand before each other like two mirrors put parallel to each other.

Unlike their western counter-parts, Indian philosophies do not present in depth analysis of human mind because mind in itself is not the end in our systems of philosophy, it is just a means.

This leads us to the question of relationship of soul with the sense-organs. In the Philosophical system as postulated by **Kapila** and **Patanjali**, their relationship is established through the doctrine of *chitchhayapatti, i.e.*, the *Purusha* casts his shadow in *Buddhi,* which is inanimate. Because of the shadow Purusha, it is activated starts working like animate.

Thus a unique relationship is presumed between *Purusha* and his counterparts in the system as envisaged by Kapila in *Samkhya* and Patanjali in *Yoga*. God is not there for granting salvation. God is not responsible for creation also. The *Samkhya* theory altogether refutes the existence of any God. Patanjali accepts a God, out defines Him as a *purusha-vis'esha.* Any *Purusha* can attain the status of God when he completely shreads off his *Klesha, karma, vipaka* and *as'aya.*

The human-being is always striving for emancipation. He is in fact always free, but finds himself captivated through this unique relationship. This system also envisages the uniqueness of the personality of each human-being. There are as many *Purushas* as the physical bodies. Each *Purusha* has to undergo through a distinct process of his own bondage and his salvation. This explains the *ad infanitum* of the process of creation and salvation. The uniqueness and distinctive nature of each personality can be explained by the example of *Ghatakas'a* as given by the author of *Yogavartika*. The *Akas'a* or ether is one and the single, but it gathers multiple forms through the contact of different objects. The *akas'a* which circumscribed within a *ghata* or pitcher is *Ghatakas'a*. It is different from the akas'a within another pitcher. In the same way each *Purusha* within his own body and sense-organs is unique and distinct from the other *purushas*.

The continuous flow of *Cittavrttis* also provides distinctive features to a human personality. The consciousness as created by the so-called unique relationship between *purusha* and *Prakriti* is viewed by the author of **Vyasabhshya** as a river, which is always flowing, it flows for the sins and it flows for **the pious.** *(Ibid., p. 4).*

Down below in this stream of consciousness, lies the mysterious world of passions and desires, of complexes and egos and libidos, which the modern Psychology terms as the subconscious. A very subtle and minute analysis of this stream of consciousness or *Chittanadi* is the mark of Patanjala Yoga system. There are five Bhumis in this stream or *chittanadi–ksipta, mudha, viksipta, ekagra* and *niruddha*. The first one is dominated by *Rajoguna*, the second one by *tamoguna*. Only the last two have the quality of *sattvaguna*. *Citta* or consciousness regains its pure form through three *shilas, viz.–prakhya, pravrtti and sthiti.*

The permutations or combinations of the types of *bhumis* and *shilas* with the *chittavrittis* lead to the formations of different type personalities. Spranger has envisaged six type of personalities. They are–Theoretical, Economic, Aesthetic, Social, Political and Religious. The persons coming under the first and the last categories can be said to be having *sattva* as a predominant quality; whereas the persons coming under the other categories may be dominated by *Rajoguna.*

Of the two types of personalities described by **Jung**, namely, extrovert and introvert, the former can be dominated by *rajoguna*, while the latter may have the prominence of *Sattvaguna*. ***Jung*** also says that the introvert type of persons try to achieve harmony in their inner world. This to a certain extant reaches near to the concept of *chittabhumis* which have *sattvaguna* in proximity.

Thus the uniqueness of human personalities is not only explained in Patanjali's system by the chain of reflection and counter reflection which connects *purusha* and *prakriti*, the system also envisages its own psycho-analytical methods and various categories to describe human personality in its own term. This description can be made very exhaustive and authentic through the following attributes–

Chittavrttis–Pramana, Viparyaya, Vikalpa etc.

Kleshas–*Avidya, Asmita, Raga, Dvesha* and *Abhinivesha.*

Vikshepas–*Vyadhi, styana, sams'aya, pramada, alasya, avirati, bhranti etc.*

Personality is in fact macrocasm in microcasm. The system as envisaged by Patanjali presents it in its immense potential. The physical body is not neglected, because, it is the very base for development of the personality. There is a concept of *Kayasampat* in Patanjali **(Yogasutra, 3.46)**. The *kayasampat* consists of *rupa, lavanya, bala* and *vajrasamhananatva*. Thus the physical beauty, grandeur and power are naturally acquired by a yogi. But is not supposed to take them as aims. They can be just the means.

The whole concept of personality as envisaged in Patanjali's system is testified by modern scientific discoveries about chromosomes and genes. Patanjali accepts the existence of *samskaras* and *vasanas* that are acquired form previous births. Consciousness is flowing for ever and in the process of continuous flow, it acquires, retains or consumes several memories, instincts and impulses which remain dormant within and are awakened on a suitable occasion.

In fact Patanjali's Yoga presents a comprehensive view of human personality, and a sound vision as well as scientific scheme for its development and emancipation.

Philosophical Approaches of Yoga

S.B. Mishra

Peace Chant of Kena Upanishad very well elaborates the aim of human existence. It declares: Om! May My Limbs, Speech, Eyes, Ears, Strength, and All My Senses Develop and Be Nourished. All This is Brahman of the Upanishads.

"May I Never Deny Brahman, May Brahman Never Deny Me. May I and Brahman be Inseparably United; May We Both be United, May All the virtues Revealed in the Upanishads Abide in Me. Who are Devoted to the Self. May they Abide in Me! Om Peace, Peace, Peace."

Every religion has tried to depict the glorious inner nature of man in various ways. The Biblical statements–**"God created man in His own Image;" The Kingdom of Heaven is within thee;"** the declaration of the Koran, the holy scripture of the Mohammedans–**"Man is a ray of God;"** and the Upanishadic statement–**"Thou art that–Tat twam Asi–**, these constitutes the basic theme of the world's religions.

Christ, Buddha, Ram, Krishna, Moses and Mohammed all spoke of the possibility of rising beyond that narrow confines of the mind in order to experience the joy and the expansion of peace in being reunited with the Divine Self. That is the goal of yoga. That is the goal of life–Self realization.

Yoga is a universal science. It is a system of philosophy promoting theory as well as practice. It is not confined to any belief, dogma or religion. It is not related to any country or faith. It is application to all people of all religions and countries.

Law of gravitation or theory of relativity was discovered by scientist who followed a particular faith or religion; but as the laws discovered by them has universal application. Similarly science of yoga was expounded by sages of India but it is relevant to all. Any one who is interested in discovering his own hidden potential and wants to evolve himself is a yoga sadhak or yogi.

Yoga is a Philosophy in Broader Sense

Philosophy is a Sanskrit term that means–"**Darshan.**" It implies to see truth for oneself. So any movement that enables a person to see the reality for himself is a philosophy. In this respect yoga is a philosophy because it presents a plan for Self realization in most effective and profound way. Adopting the principles and practices of yoga teachings one can realize his essential nature directly. In this way it may be called as a Darshan.

Philosophical Approaches of Yoga

Different philosophical approaches of yoga are based on profound study of human personality. One can realize his essential nature on following four planes:

1. Plane of Action
2. Plane of Emotion
3. Plane of Will and
4. Plane of Wisdom. (slide aspects of personality)

These are also four basic tendencies through which one expresses himself and communicate with others. Yoga has adopted each of these as a potent means for Selfrealisation there by presenting following four major paths:

1. Karma Yoga for Action
2. Bhakti Yoga for Emotion
3. Raja Yoga for Will and
4. Jnana Yoga for Perfection of Wisdom aspect of personality.

Once there is complete evolution of these four foundations of human personality one can realize his essential nature to be universal Self underlying entire creation. He then discovers that he is not a limited individual but **Brahman**–the Absolute.

The Best Path

Although any of the four paths described above is capable of leading one to the highest goal of the Self realization; but the best approach prescribed by yoga is the synthesis of all the four which is called **Integral Yoga.** It combines the principles and practice of all yogas in daily life. This is safe, sure and steady process to achieve the highest objective of life.

Integral yoga presents unique approach which is most effective, practical and universally accepted. There is nothing to lose. One can evolve while experiencing this world and enjoying it with detached attitude.

Yoga is a Process of Constant Adjustment with Cosmic Harmony

During the state of harmony and integration, the human personality is tuned to the cosmic unity which permeates the entire creation. **(slide sheath of body)**

At no level of existence, can one separate oneself from the universal unity of existence. The physical sheath is a wave of the ocean of material energy. Every thing belongs to cosmic life. Similarly the vital sheath is a wave of the cosmic prana. The mental sheath is a radiation of the cosmic mind. The intellectual sheath is an emanation of the universal mind-stuff. The very individual soul is a reflection of the cosmic spirit–the Atman.

The ego-center which perceives "mine" and "thine" in conjuction with a limited mind is the basis of the illusory individualized existence. If the vision is led beyond the ego by the practice of enquiry and profound reflection on the nature of the innermost self, one would experience the unity of universal life to which all beings and all objects, form parts of one organic whole.

An aspirant delights in practising this stupendous adjustment with the cosmos in every part of his personality. It is this process of constant adjustment which assumes different names, such as **Jnana yoga** wherein the reason adjusts with cosmic intuition, **Bhakti yoga** for the feelings aspect of personality to commune with the universal harmony, **Raja yoga** for the will to become a channel of the cosmic will, so that the mind unruffled by thoughts and desires may reflect the nature of the Self and **Karma yoga** where the day to day activities, and the desire that sustain them are adjusted with the universal activity, where action is a recreation, a participation in universal sacrifice, and a process of spiritual transformation leading to Self-realization.

Yoga always advocates all sided development, a complete integration of personality. There is no need to be over enthusiastic for attaining Self realization, there is no need to over stress one aspect of personality, in order to move towards the Self. The process of spiritual attainment is characterised by spontaneity, grace, smoothness, and silence.

The ringing bell of yoga inspires us to be ever awake. Be ever alive. Be ever active. Be vibrant with cosmic light, love, and action. Experience the joys of detachment. Feel the strength of increasing wisdom. Float on the ocean on divine feeling, soar in the infinite realms of liberation. Thus, one attains Self realization wherein he becomes the one with the all.

Historical Perspectives on Yoga

M.L. Gharote

Introduction

The origin of Yoga is obscured in its great antiquity. No systematic study recording development of Yoga through its evolutionary stages has been undertaken so far. Historically what we know about Yoga is very little. It is a gigantic task to understand the systematic development and various progressive stages of development of Yoga.

In order to take a brief survey of the historical development of Yoga based on the available sources and Yogic literature we may consider the different periods of history as follows:

1. Prevedic Period
2. Vedic Period
3. Upanisadic Period
4. Epic Period
5. Sutra Period
6. Smriti Period
7. Pauranic Period
8. Medieval Period
9. Modern Period

1. Prevedic Period

From the excavation of the Indus Valley we find that Yoga in some form was practised during that period. The idol of Mother

Goddess and the figure seated in the Yogic posture suggest the antiquity of Yoga. Some believe that Yoga owes much to the pre-Aryan heritage.

2. Vedic Period

Although scholars differ in their opinion about the connection of Indus Valley civilization with Vedic civilization the source of Yoga is undoubtedly found in the Vedic literature. In Vedas we find the description of mystic experiences. Certain concepts of Yoga which were developed later are seen in their rudimentary form in Vedas. But it is surprising to note that the words Yoga and Yogis are not used in their technical sense in Vedas.

The word 'Yoga is used in Ṛgveda in quite a different sense. It has come in the sense of 'Yoking' of the horses to the chariot or in the sense of 'connection'.

At another place it denotes 'acquiring the unacquired'. However, Yoga as an end of acquiring tranquility of mind or samadhi is nowwhere clearly mentioned in the Ṛgveda. This suggests that Yoga did not attain its technical meaning during the Vedic times. The word 'Yogi'–the practitioner of Yoga is conspicuously absent in Ṛgveda. In the sense of 'Yogis' other words such as Munis, Manishine, Ṛsis, Kavis, Kosins, Vzatyns (in Atharveda) have been used. The 'Muni sukta' of Ṛgveda points out to the existence of a class of people similar to Yogis.

The concept of Prana in Yoga as the dynamic life principle can be traced is the Atharva Veda. The words 'Prāṇati' and 'Apānati' used suggest the concepts of Prāṇa and Apāna. Thus, though the fully grown system of Yoga is not found in Vedic Period, origin of several Yogic concepts could be traced in Vedic literature.

We find the growth of certain Yogic tenets in the Brāhmaṇas like Satapatha, Aitareya, Kausitaki, Jaiminiya and Gopatha. In these we get elaborate description of Prāṇavidyā and advanced ideas regarding Praṇava Vidyā. Praṇava is another technical name for OM. Brāhmaṇa literature mainly represents the further development of ritualism of Vedas. Different Brāhmaṇas have been affiliated to the different Vedas. S'atapatha Brahmana is the largest and most important Brahmana.

3. Upanishadic Period

Real basis for the system of Yoga can be found in the Upanishads. Marliest Upanishads like Chhāndogya and Brihadāraṇyaka give us the basis of Kriyāyoga. But the words Yoga and Yogin are not found in their technical sense. Prāṇa and Nāḍis are important topics discussed there. In Kaṭhopnishad the word Yoga has been used in its technical sense. In the three Upanisads, namely, Is'a, Kena and Kaṭha we see the formation of firm basis of Yoga. The Shvetāshvatara in perhaps most important from Yogic point of view. It describes sequence of Yogic practises and their physiological effects. Its tradition is seen continued in the later Haṭha texts. The two prose Upanisads, namely, Aitareya and Taittirīya describe different Kos'as of the body.

4. Epic Period

The two great Indian epics, namely, Rārāyaṇa and Mahābhārata are the rich source of information about various kinds of Yogic practices prevalent then. Yoga as a system seems to be quite popular in the age of Rāmāyaṇa. The most important section dealing with Yoga in Mahābhārata is the famous Bhagawadgītā. It deals with the characteristics of the realised Yogin and the three paths of Yoga, namely, Jñāna, Bhakti and Karma. It is a synthesis of various ideas and practices of Yoga.

From ancient times a number of commentaries have been written on Bhagawadgītā and several critical studies, commentaries and translations are published every year. It is translated in all the world languages.

3. Sūtra Period

Patanjali's Yogasūtras are the oldest systematic treatise on Yoga available to us. It contains 195 aphorisms divided into 4 chapters. It is based on the previous and contemporary traditions of Yoga and has exerted a great influence on later thinkers and practitioners of Yoga. Several commentaries have been written on the Yogasūtras of Patañjali. These throw light on the development of different Yogic concepts and techniques of that period. The first commentary on Yogasūtras is known as Vyāsabhāsya. The sutras would have remained altogether unintelligible without this Vyāsabhāṣya.

The Vyāsabhāṣya again has been commented upon by several writers like on Śaṅkarācharya (not the famous exponent of Vedanta School), Vacaspati Miśra of Tattvaviaśāradi, Bhojarāja of Vṛttis, Vijñānabhikṣu of Yogavārtika, Bhāvā Gaṇeśa and Nāgoji bhatta. Besides these, there are commentaries by Nārāyaṇatīrtha, Rāmānandayati, Anantadeva and Hariprasāda. Among recent commentaries are those of Bālārāma Udāsīna, Baldev Miśra and Hariharānanda Āraṇya. There are also some commentaries published in regional languages of India. Some good English translations with comments are now available.

Among the unpublished commentaries may be mentioned those of Gopāla, Bhavadeva, Sīmananda, Ānandasiṣya, Udayankara, Umāpati Tripāṭhi, Jñānānanda, Mahādeva, Rāmānuja, Vṛndāvana Śukla, Rāghavānanda and Śridhara.

Buddhism

Buddhism has been greatly influenced by Yoga and it has also contributed a great deal to the development of Yoga. Buddha himself had practised Yoga under the teachers Arada Kalam and Uddaka Ramaputta.

There are striking similarities of concepts and terms in early Buddhist scriptures and yogasūtras of Patañjali which have given rise to the problem of relative priority of the Buddhist or the Pātañjala Yoga.

The fourfold dhyāna referred to by early Buddhist scriptures is one of the significant contributions to Yoga. In Yogasūtras of Patañjali also almost the same scheme is discussed. Besides the fourfold dhyāna, in Buddhist texts are described the four Brahmavihāras of sublime occupations–cultivating four exalted psychological moods which are:

(1) Love (Maitri), (2) Compassion (Karaṇā), (3) Cheerfulness (Muditā), and (4) Indifference (Upekṣā).

Following are some remarkable resemblances between Pātañjala Yoga System and early Buddhist Yoga.

(i) Both accept the four noble truths and emphasize that Yoga removes misery.

(ii) Both do not consider the absolute necessity of Godhead. Buddha is silent while according to Patanjali it is one of the alternative paths.

(iii) Both accept the concept of Samādhi.

(iv) There is ideological and terminological similarity between Nirvāṇa.

(v) There is a parallelism in using eightfold path of Yoga.

This similarity has given rise to the problem of relative priority of the Buddhist or the Pātañjala Yoga. It is possible that both may have a common source wherefrom they have borrowed.

Later Buddhism was divided into different sects and Buddhist Yoga grow in several branches. Most of them belong to the post-Patañjali Period.

Jainism

Mahāvīra the founder of Jainism was a contemporary of Gautam Buddha and was undoubtedly a great practical Yogi. Mahāvīra is considered to be the twenty fourth prophet in the Jain tradition. Unfortunately, no early works of the Jain prophets are available today.

Yoga according to Jain tradition also consists in Yoking body, speech, and mind. It is called Upayoga. Jains speak of the threefold Yoga–Jñāna Yoga, Ischā Yoga and Kriyā Yoga. Much of the Jain teachings resemble those of Bhagawad Gītā. Jainism accepts correct outlook (Samyog darśana), Correct knowledge (Samyog caritra) together as the path of liberation.

For the correct conduct Jain texts prescribe certain vows to be observed to the best of one's capacity in the beginning and then to be observed absolutely. The early prophets have prescribed non-violence, truth, non-stealing and continence. It is believed that Mahavira added non-possession as the fifth vow. These vows are just the same as Patanjali has included within Yama, the first step of eightfold Yoga. Patanjali might have borrowed this from Jainism including the term Mahāvrata meaning absolute vow.

Meditation resulting in liberation in Jainism is said to be fourfold: Righteous meditation, auspicious meditation, white meditation, and pure meditation. It is probable that Patanjali might have added Jain meditation at the end of the third chapter of Yogasūtras.

The available works on Jainism are of post-Patanjali period. There are several later works by Jain authors dealing with different types and aspects of Yoga written under the influence of Patanjalis Yogasūtras and Hathayoga. Some of the important ones may be mentioned as 'Yoga-śāstra by Hemacandra with his own commentary on it, Yogabindu, Pravacanasāra, Yogadṛṣṭi-samuccaya, Yogasāra, Paramātmaprakāśa. Tattvārthādhigamasūtra, Ācārāṅga, Uttarādhyayana.

6. Smriti Period

The period of Smriti literature starts from the times of Patanjali. Some Smrities had been composed before 500 B.C. and they were written till about 1000 A.D. During this long period of smriti literature we find the changes in the prevailing ideas, beliefs, worships and customs. The Smrities tried to combine Yoga with the daily rituals. Thus we find Pranayama and certain purificatory technique occupying important place in every ritual. A collection of 27 Smrities is available in print. One of the important older Smrities, namely, Brihadyogīyājñavalkya Smriti has been critically edited and published by the Kaivalyudhama, Lonavla.

7. Pauranic Stage

The Purāṇas are a class of literature which existed from very ancient times. The extant Purāṇas are recaste made of the ancient Purānas during the first century of the Christian era.

The orthodox number of Puranas is 18 which may be mentioned as follows:

(1) Brahma, (2) Padma, (3) Visnu, (4) Vayu, (5) Bhagavata, (6) Naradiya, (7) Markandeya, (8) Agni, (9) Bhavisya, (10) Brahma-Vaivarta, (11) Linga, (12) Varaha, (13) Skanda, (14) Vamana, (15) Kurma, (16) Matsya, (17) Caruda, and (18) Brahmanda.

Many of these Puranas deal with the Yogangas. Some of them also describe the Yogicarya (conduct of a Yogi). The Vayu, Brahmanda, Matsya and Visnu are probably the eldest among the extent Puranas. From time to time Puranas received substantial additions.

There are also 18 Upapuranas. Although there is no uniformity in the enumeration of the Upapuranas the following names may be mentioned:

(1) Sanatkumara, (2) Narasimha, (3) Nanda, (4) Sivadharma, (5) Durvasa, (6) Naradiya, (7) Kapila, (8) Vamana, (9) Usanas, (10) Mgnava, (11) Varuna, (12) Kali, (13) Mahesvara, (14) Samba, (15) Saura, (16) Parasara, (17) Marica, and (18) Bhargava.

The number of Upapuranas is much more–even to the extent of hundred; but hardly 15 have been printed. The nature of Upapuranas is sectarian and the philosophy and practices of different sects are usually described in these.

8. Medieval Period

Tantar Stage–There is a vast literature on Tantras published and unpublished. There are Buddhist Tantras, Hindu Tantras and Jain Tantras. Tantras are commonly associated by Shakti-worship, with mudras, mantras, mandalas, the five Makaras, the Dakshinamarga, Vama-marga, and Magic practices for acquiring supernatural powers. It is difficult to say which Tantras are earlier. There are very large number of subjects included in the Tantras. Buddhist and Hindu Tantras have great resemblance, although they differ in the topics discussed. Many of the tantra works were introduced in Tibet, China, Japan and South East Asia. Many of the original Sanskrit works are not now available although translations of some of them are available in Tibetan. Seventh to twelfth century was the period of Tantrik works and cults, both Hindu and Buddhist. The Tantrikas substituted a Yoga of enjoyment for the Yoga of abstience and asceticism. The Tantras claim that liberation is achieved by the very means by which otherwise one falls. The Tantras tried to differentiate three dispositions of 'Pasubhava (animal disposition), 'Virabhava (heroic disposition), and 'Divyabhava (divine disposition) which are graded according to the nature and stage of the practicants. It is in the final disposition that the practicant rises above sense enjoyment altogether.

Natha Cult–Tantrism developed into Rajayoga and Sahajayana of Buddhist. Rajayoga is very much confused with Patanjali's Yoga.

As an aid to Rajayoga Hathayoga was evolved and became very popular through the Natha Cult. Many of the Hathayogic practices seem to have their origin in Tantrism. Nathayoga laid a great emphasis on preparing the body as a vehicle for attaining the higher spiritual experiences. It is this yoga which has become so popular throughout the world. Some of the traditional and important texts may be mentioned as 'Siddha-siddhanta Paddhati', 'Goraksa Sataka', 'Hatha Pradipika', 'Gheranda Samhita', 'Siva Samhita'.

Many other texts are as yet in manuscript form awaiting publication. Out of these a few could be named as 'Hatha Ratnavali', 'Hathasamkata candrika', 'Yoga cintamini' etc. Kaivalyadhama, Lonavla is publishing an exhaustive catalogue of Yoga manuscripts deposited in several libraries. This will provide a wealth of information of the Yoga literature in more recent times.

Bhakti Cult

Yoga also had its impacts on Bhakti literature. The saints have profusely written on Bhakti and depending on their background they refer to yoga practices now and then. The Bhagawata Purana is looked upon as a bible by the Vaisnavita sect. The Sandilyasutras and Naradasutras deal systematically with different aspects of Bhakti.

9. Modern Period

Unless we refer to development of Yoga in modern times the survey of historical development of Yoga would not be complete. The tradition of Yoga continues even today without break. In modern times Swami Vivekananda made Yoga popular. Swami Ramtirtha and Paramahansa Yogananda continued his work to spread the knowledge of Yoga out of India. Raman Maharshi, Sri Aurobindo and Swami Shivananda of Rishikesh are some other names of modern exponents.

Swami Kuvalayananda made the scientific aspect of Yoga popular. He pointed out on the basis of scientific evidence how yoga could be useful in our day to day life.

Conclusion

Yoga has always remained a growing discipline and has adjusted to the needs of the day. It never prescribed the same approach to everyone. It always had the regard for individual differences. This special feature of yoga will also govern the trend of future developments in Yoga. This invariably will involve the applied aspect which we see very popular today.

The Philosophy of Yoga

K.P. Nath

Yoga is one of the six systems of ancient Indian philosophy. It is a Sanskrit work derived form its root verb 'yuj' meaning to unite or to yoke. Yoga is its noun form and means union. It is concerned with the union of the individual soul with the Absolute or the Divine soul. Maharshi Patanjali, believed to be living in the 2nd Century B.C., is the founder of this school of philosophical thought. The Yoga Sutra, a treatise written by him collecting materials scattered in the Vedas and the Upanishads, provides the basis of this philosophy. As a philosophical thought, it comes very close to the Sankhya school of Indian philosophy which considers all materials beings, both animate and inanimate, in the universe, as 'prakriti' and an all pervading superconscious spirit as 'purusha'. Buddhism as a philosophical thought outside the six well-defined schools of Indian philosophy has much affinity with Yoga in that both speak of non-violence, non-appropriation, non-attachment, austerities like living on the barest minimum necessities, concentration and meditation as pre-requisites leading to their respective goals. While for Yoga, the goal is the conscious union of the individual soul with the Supreme soul during one's present life itself, for Buddhism, it is avoidance of the cycle of birth and rebirth and attainment of 'nirvana' or salvation after death. While Yoga provides eight-fold steps in sequential order to be followed for the blissful union with the Divine, Buddhism provides eight noble paths to be followed to avoid rebirth.

The beatitude of God realisation can be experienced in any of the principally four different yogic ways–through Bhakti or devotion, through 'niskama karma' or detached labour, through 'jnana' or knowledge and also through meditation, often called the Raja Yoga.

In Bhakti Yoga, the devotee surrenders himself completely before the Divine and intensely aspires to get merged with Him. Widespread appeal of Bhakti Yoga is manifest in many religions. An element of simplicity of heart and emotional upsurge are the characteristic marks of Bhakti Yoga. It appeals to the common unlettered people who do not apply their sense of reasoning and, therefore, can surrender before the Divine will completely. Bhakti dissolves the ego and purifies the heart, as one-pointed devotion takes away all the impurities of the heart like lust, anger, greed, pride, jealousy, hatred and deceit and such other baser emotions. Bhakti requires simplicity of heart and intense devotion. Reason and intellect as provided by education has nothing to do with the Bhakti way.

In Karma Yoga, karma or work, when performed with whole-hearted attention but with complete detachment, can also lead an individual to the blissful state of the mind. To a karma yogi, no work is considered small or mean. Many great saints and sages of the past had chosen works for their livelihood that might be considered base or ignoble in the opinion of an ordinary man. Kabir was a weaver and Rabidas used to mend shoes. God remains with those who work. The Bible also enjoins, "Man shall live by the sweat of his brow." Karma Yoga is the Yoga of action. Karma when done with detachment brings poise to the spirit. Karma Yoga is seen at the finest in the life of many great men. Mahatma Gandhi exemplified Karma Yoga by spinning.

Jnana Yoga is meant for the highly rational and intellectually gifted individuals engaged in the task of acquiring knowledge and gaining wisdom. When wisdom is attained, ignorance encircling the inner self in thick layers falls off layer by layer releasing the soul from its bondage. Ignorance encages the soul and renders it dull and dead; knowledge brings it back to its vivacious and effulgent state. It emancipates the mind from all baser emotions and develops a feeling of detachment about worldly matters like the desire for name, fame, power and possession and turns the mind towards the Divine Spirit. Thus when ignorance vanishes from the mind, the liberated mind creates a conducive ambience for the individual soul to merge with the Supreme soul.

The Raja Yoga provides an ordered sequence of practices starting from Yama (moral restraints) and Niyama (observances) through Asana (body posture) and Pranayama (breath control), Pratyahara (sense abstraction), Dharana (concentration) and Dhyana (meditation) culminating into the final stage called Samadhi (superconscious bliss), a state where individual soul mingles with the Supreme soul as a river merges into the ocean to lose its identity. Raja Yoga is the king of all Yogas and as such is often called the Royal Yoga. Raja Yoga is mainly concerned with meditation so as to achieve ultimately the state of Samadhi, the blissful union with the Divine. Therefore, it stresses upon the last four steps of Yoga beginning with Pratyahara followed by Dharana as preparatory steps to mediation. However, in Raja Yoga, the first four steps beginning with Yama followed by Niyama, Asana and Pranayama are also important and cannot be neglected in disciplining body, mind and spirit so as to be able to achieve perfection in all the rest foursteps. Asana and Pranayama alone considered together constitute, what is called, Hatha Yoga and have gained world-wide acceptance because of their beneficial effect on body, mind and spirit.

Raja Yoga is in fact the Yoga proper and, therefore, unless otherwise stated, the word Yoga usually refers to Raja Yoga. However, because of its world-wide popularity, Hatha Yoga nowadays has come to be synonymous with Yoga. Raja Yoga has eight well-defined steps as stated before. These are called the eight limbs of Yoga. Raja Yoga is, therefore, often called Astanga Yoga, 'asta' means eight and 'anga' means limbs. These are elaborated below:

Yama refers to moral restraint and consists of five moral codes of conduct. These are Ahimsa or non-violence, Satya or truthfulness, Asteya or non-stealing, Brahmacharya or continence and Aparigraha or non-coveting. Non-violence is the first pre-requisite to Yama. The principle of non-injury is to be observed. One must refrain from causing harm to others. Even displaying anger and speaking sharply and reprovingly tantamounts to violence. There must be compassion, love and regard not only for one's fellow men but for animals and small creatures as well. One must be truthful in thought, word and deed. One must not steal. Lying and stealing have corrupting effect on the mind. They vilify the spirit. One must also cultivate continence avoiding undue indulgence in sexual pleasures. One must not also covet. Adherence to these moral restraints keeps the mind free from cares, worries and anxieties. A cool, calm, quiet and composed mind that ensues is conducive to spiritual realisation which is the ultimate objective of Yoga.

Niyama provides another five principles for observation to fortify the five moral codes prescribed under Yama. These are Saucha or cleanliness, Santosha or contentment, Tapas or hardihood, Swadhyaya or self-study of sacred books and Iswar Pranidhana or devotion to God. One must be clean both physically and mentally. One must develop a sense of contentment, a feeling of satisfaction in all situations of life. One must practise austerities or hardihood discarding all sorts of luxuries and comfort and by living with the barest minimum necessities. It includes all austerities like fasting once a fortnight, sleeping on hare bed, walking barefooted, keeping silence, minimising sleep, eating modest meal, maintaining strict routine of work, avoiding sloth and such other rigours. Tapas is like a blazing fire that brings lusters in the life of an individual. Regular study of sacred books uplifts the mind by filling it with noble thoughts. Self-surrender to the Lord removes egotism, pride, vanity and all such impurities from the mind. Yama and Niyama are complementary concepts. Both together prepare an individual for the onward stages of Yoga.

Asana refers to various body postures. Because of their popularity, Yoga has become synonymous with these body postures. Asanas are meant for keeping the body supple and flexible, agile and young. Asanas not only increase the flexibility of various body limbs but also enhance the beauty of the body by reducing disproportionate accumulation of fat in the body. Asanas also have beneficial effects on the spinal cord of the body. It is said in Yoga, "You are as young as your spine is young." Asanas in particular help correct deformities in the spine. They also activate the central nervous system of the brain and the peripheral nervous system in the body, help proper blood circulation, tone up the sagging muscles and make the body free from disease. As Asanas improve both physical and mental health, they have been provided a very prominent place in Yoga. The main objective of Asanas is to make the body fit for prolonged sitting in silent meditation.

Pranayama refers to the art and science of correct breathing. In Yoga philosophy, fresh air has been recognised as 'prana', the elan vital or the life-sustaining energy. It consists in devices by which the best can be achieved out of breathing. It emphasizes upon deep rhythmic breathing in place of the shallow and irregular ones. Pranayama helps take out waste metabolism from inside the body in the form of carbondioxide most effectively and thus helps the heart function efficiently. Pranayama practices are complimentary to the Asana practices. When performed together, they ensure sound physical and mental health. A person with the regular habit of practising various Asanas and Pranayamas can live easily upto one hundred years and even beyond. 'Satayurboi manushya', so proclaims the Yoga Sutra. Besides providing longevity to life, both Asana and Pranayama prepare the body and mind to enter to inner circle of Yoga which starts with Pratyahara.

Pratyahara refers to sense withdrawal. Physical senses continuously react to the vast array of stimuli in the environment. It affects the concentration of mind. Pratyahara or the abstraction of senses is the initial step towards total mastery over the senses. In Pratyahara, the senses no longer respond to the external cues that hinder mental concentration. Sense abstraction is an arduous practice and requires intense endeavour on the part of an aspirant of Yoga to master it. The practice of sense withdrawal develops in the Yoga aspirant control over the sense organs and helps his mental concentration. Pratyahara or his withdrawal of the senses is often compared to the drawing of various limbs of a tortoise within its shell.

Dharana refers to the concentration of mind which has the tendency to get scattered like a fistful of mustard seeds when placed on a sheet of paper. But if the scattered mind can be brought under control and firmly set to one focal point, concentration is said to be achieved. Generally, the centre of the forehead or navel or a pointed source of a soothing light at a distance is the object where the mind is sought to be fixed. Concentration of mind provides one poise and placidity, the precondition for meditation. Concentration is a matter of practice spread over a period of time. Beside facilitating meditation, concentration improves mental abilities of imagining, perceiving, thinking and remembering.

Dhyana literally means meditation sitting with a cool, collected, composed and concentrated mind. Meditation is a state of mind where it has ceased wandering and has become steadfast with one and only one idea. It is process that leads one the innermost recess of the mind to bring one face to face with the truth one may be searching for. Prolonged meditation leads one to self-realisation by gradually removing the outer layers of illusion which shrouds the truth. Dhyana is an essential prelude to Samadhi, the last stage of Yoga.

Samadhi is the final stage of Yoga in which the mind transcends the physical senses and full spiritual consciousness is attained. It is a state of blissful union of the individual soul with the Supreme soul which is the ultimate goal of Yoga. When this goal is achieved, the Yogi becomes conscious of the Absolute in him. He loses all sense of self, circumstances and sensation and becomes completely absorbed in the Supreme. It is a state of ecstasy, a state of supreme bliss. In this state, the individual consciously achieves the Divine in him or he can be said to have been merged with the Divine. It is often compared to the merging of a river with the ocean, where the river loses its identity and becomes one with the ocean. Individual soul and the Supreme soul blend harmoniously in that state of total bliss known as 'kaivalya'.

Sense withdrawal, concentration, meditation and Samadhi, the state of total bliss are, in fact, one continuous process, each being a step leading directly to the next. These four are also purely mental processes, whereas the preceding four, *viz,* moral restraints, observances, body postures and breath regulation, refer to physical processes meant for preparing the body to make it a fit vehicle to enter the rest four steps of Yoga. The eight stages of Yoga in ordered sequence also form complementary pairs. The first two, *viz.*, Yama and Niyama are complementary to each other as also the third and the fourth, *viz.*, Asana and Pranayama, fifth and sixth, *viz.*, Pratyahara and Dharana, and the seventh and the eighth, *viz.*, Dhyana and Samadhi. A Yoga aspirant has to master sequentially all the eight stages in order to be able to attain the blissful state of Samadhi. There is no substitute of Yoga for acquiring the equanimity of the mind.

Yoga is both an intellectual system and a practical means to achieve inner harmony. Despite its philosophical underpinnings, Yoga is primarily a pragmatic discipline. Yoga is both a science and a philosophy, a science its tenets have been proved true through practice, and a philosophy because it speaks of realms beyond the scope of science. Through Yoga is considered one of the six systems on Indian philosophy and sometimes referred to as the Patanjala Darsan, according to many philosophers, it primarily stands for a body of practical disciplines rather than any philosophical theory proper.[1]

Yoga is rooted to India's hoary past. Archeological evidence shows that Yoga was practised in India prior to 2000 B.C. by the inhabitants of the Indus Valley.[2] With the arrival of the Aryans in India shortly after 2000 B.C., the principles of Yoga came to be recorded in scattered forms in Sanskrit, an Indo-European language, in their sacred books–the Vedas and the Upanishads. Yoga as an organised study of its principles and practices took shape and emerged as a philosophical system from the basic Upanishadic teachings around 2nd Century B.C. like all the other Indian philosophies.

Yoga is a subject of such breadth and depth that it covers every possible phase of human existence. The fact that it has existed unchanged for so many years, speaks clearly of its veracity and usefulness to mankind. Truth must always stand unchanged for it is factual and cannot be modified.[3]

Though the subject-matter of Yoga has been taken from the sacred books of the Hindus, by itself Yoga is not a religion, for it is bereft of any rites or rituals, doctrines or dogmas, creeds or cults as in religions. Its teachings are so basic and fundamental that there is practically no religion or creed to which its aims and objectives are contradictory or antagonistic. Indeed, adherents to any religion, or even those who profess no religious beliefs at all, can find beneficence in Yoga. It is interesting to note that a most useful book called Christian Yoga has been written by a Catholic Jesuit, Father J.M. Dechanel, in which the practice of Yoga has been recommended as an aid to Christianity.[4]

Practically, Yoga, as it is taught today, is based on the Sutras of Patanjali, and it is a fact that the teachings remain practically unchanged, as they were originally in the Vedas and the Upanishads, even though many years have passed, many generations of thinkers and philosophers have come and gone and man in general has developed considerably in the mean time. The teachings of Yoga are, therefore, timeless and are as right and effective today as they were thousands of Year ago.[5]

In the past, treatises on Yoga were available only in Sanskrit, a language taught only to the upper castes, and every effort was taken to protect its knowledge to prevent it from falling into wrong hands. Nowadays, however, the language is taught is quite openly and books on Yoga have been widely translated and published. Schools of Yoga are now well established not only in India but in many parts of the world including America and Europe attracting sincere students of all races and religions, creeds and climes learning Yoga under expert Yoga teachers. Besides a host of centres of Yoga studies as exists on both sides of the Atlantic, the London School of Yoga and the American Academy of Asian Studies are engaged in the study of and experimentation with Yoga. In the world-wide increasing popularity of Yoga alone lies the ample proof of its efficacy in providing a healthy, happy and harmonious living.

In the residential schools inside deep forests maintained by the sages of ancient India, the disciples were required to observe the principles of Yoga during their life lived with the preceptor in his 'ashrama'. This is because Yoga philosophy provides certain principles of life that have been considered essential for the development of the complete man, which is the ultimate aim of all education. Yoga provides an excellent means for the development of body, mind and spirit. This is the reason why great emphasis was laid for the Yogic way of life among the disciples in the system of education that prevailed in ancient India. Even to this day, physical, mental and spiritual well-being has been considered supreme in all education without which education is considered meaningless. Mahatma Gandhi in our day has considered education as one that develops body, mind and spirit. Yoga philosophy has provided a principle of life that has aimed towards achieving physical, mental and spiritual well-being, a principle that has withstood the test of time and place, the hallmark of any true philosophy. More so, Yoga stands on the dividing line of both science and philosophy as the science of all sciences and the philosophy of all philosophies.

References

1. Chatterjee, D.P., Indian Philosophy, People's Publishing House, New Delhi, 1964, p.31.
2. Mayo, DeBarra, Yoga Book II, Runner's World Books, Anderson World Books, Inc.,1400 Stierlin Road, Mountain View, CA 94043, 1983, p.14.
3. McCartney, James, Yoga : The Key to life, Jaico Publishing House, Bombay, 1970, p.6.
4. *Ibid.*, p.7.
5. *Ibid.*, p.5.

Bibliography for further studies

Bernard, Thoes, Heaven Lies Within Us, Rider, London.

Brunton, Paul, The Secret Path, Rider, London.

Dechanel, J.M., Christian Yoga, Burnes & Oates, London.

Dunne, Desmond, The Easy Way to Go, Panther Books, London.

Amaldas, Brahmachari, Yoga & Contemplation, Darton, Longman & Todd, London.

Anand, Ambar Raj, Yoga for All, New Light Publishers, New Delhi.

Desai, Morarji, Nature Cure, S. Chand & Co., New Delhi.

Devi, Indra, Forever Young, Forever Healthy, Jaico Publishing, Bombay.

Jivaka, Sramanera, Growing Up Into Buddhism, Maha Bodhi Society, Calcutta.

Joshi, K.S., Yoga in Daily Life, Orient Paperbacks, New Delhi.

Krishnananda, Swami, The Yoga System, Divine Life Society, Tehri Garhwal.

Munshi, K.M., Foundations of Indian Culture, Bharatiya Vidya Bhavan, Bombay.

Nath, Pandit Shambhu, Speaking of Yoga, Sterling Publishers, New Delhi.

Pandit, M.P., Yoga for the Modern Man, Sterling Publishers, New Delhi.

Raghavan, V. (Ed.), Founders of Philosophy, Publications Division, Govt. of India, New Delhi.

Sivananda, Swami, Practical Lessons in Yoga, Divine Life Society, Tehri Garhwal, U.P.

Sivanands, Swami, Ananda Gita, Divine Life Society, Tehri Garhwal, U.P.

Sri Aurobindo, Bases of Yoga, Sri Aurobindo Ashram, Pondicherry.

Srinivasachari, P.N., The Ethical Philosophy of the Gita, Sri Ramakrishna Math, Mylapore, Madras.

Yogendra, Shri, Facts About Yoga, The Yoga Institute, Santa Cruz, Bombay.

Yogendra, Shri, Yoga Asanas Simplified, The Yoga Institute, Santa Cruz, Bombay.

Yogendra, Sita Devi, Yoga Simplified for Women, The Yoga Institute, Santa Cruz, Bombay.

Wood, Ernest, Yoga, Penguin Books, London.

Causes of Violence and Unity of Human Consciousness : A Philosophical, Religious, Scientific and Meditational Understanding

Y.S. Vagrecha

There are *deterministic philosophies*, where cause and effect are predetermined and there is no free choice. When one is guided by such thinking in conceptualising the human nature, one is bound to generate violence. Here there is no room for hope, freedom and self actualisation. There is no scope for realising the potentialities. It is a closed world, dehumanizing world, full of atrocities and injustice. Maslow (1968) says that the process of healthy growth is a never ending series of free-choice situations: choice between safety or growth, dependence or independence, regression or progression, immaturity or maturity and so on. Not allowing people to act at their free will implies a certain lack of respect for them and for humanity in a broader sense. It is an act which tantamount to seedling of violence in them. The ancient sages have realized this fact long ago. That's why in *Upanishads* every assertion about reality is added with *neti-neti i.e.*, it is not this alone, it is not this alone, (wrongly translated as it is not this, it is not this.) a real undeterministic approach to life and a thoroughly relativistic approach to truth.

The *Mahabharata* similarly points to the other truths of every thing including 13 attributes of truth, while accepting that its limit does not end here only. However, for the first time, a more formal philosophical development of relativity of truth, carrying further the earlier concern of *Upanishads* and *Mahabharata* can be seen in *Jainism.*

Jainism does not believe absolutism in knowledge and in attitudes. A statement regarding a thing, person or situation is true only conditionally. Truth and falsehood largely depends on the standpoint from which we perceive the things. A 'Stand-point' is called *'Naya'* in *Jainism.* Logically it is connected with Jain *Syada-vada* which suggests that to every assertion one has to add a *'Syat'* or 'may be' or 'in a sense.' A thing can be perceived from at least seven different stand points *(saptabhangi-naya).* A thing can be described as existing one and can also be described as not existing one and can also be described as existing and non existing and so on. This awareness of the many sidedness of reality or truth is also known as *anekanta-vada* in *Jainism.*

Syada-Vada alongwith *anekantavada* had held that there are several different ways of perceiving reality, each valid in its own way and none of them true absolutely.

Violence in interpersonal relationships, in social and collective life and between nations is due to absolute claim for truth. When I close myself, mentally and emotionally, to the truth of another, I create the very first condition of violence. Every form of human violence (take any example) has emerged from the competing one sided notion of truth. That my truth is the truth and your truth is the falsehood, and I will force my truth upon you, if I can. Clinging unknowingly to what is partly true but believe it to be the whole truth. All clinging is *parigraha* which leads to violence, hence, the *Jaina* emphasis on *a-parigraha* or not clinging. Thus non deterministic philosophies and relativistic approach to truth liberate us from the violence of one sided truth, and strengthen the unity of human consciousness.

Every religion talk about an 'experience' whether personal, collective or cumulative in nature. But in articulating this experience, language limps and stammers. It is very difficult to express this experience in the existing vocabulary. One finds no words. To facilitate this experience to passover generations it leaps into 'Faith.' Faith is basically self-surrender in trust to the 'mystery.' Later on, through institutionalisation it easily becomes an 'ideology', that is, a set of ideas through which one can understand and control one's world and feel secure in it. Religious as well as political ideologies put forth a view of truth and a way of liberation and happiness, but their claims of absolute truth come in conflict with each other so greatly that far from bringing happiness, they bring confrontation and misery. It is ironical that nothing has separated the peoples of the world more than their respective ideas of truth through religion, ism or otherwise. We are alike when we lie, but fall apart when we talk of truth.

The *fundamentalism* has replaced the true spirit of religion and is all pervasive. It emphasise rites, rituals, scriptures, taboos rather than personalising religious experience. In the guise of religious practices it attempts to capture political power. It became a tool of dehumanisation and oppression rather than an instrument of peace and liberation. Inspite of all these dividing forces there is unity of human consciousness. Carl Gustav Jung believed this collective, universal conscious is unconscious which manifests itself through the individual mind. Acquired traits and cultural patterns are transmitted in each individual from generation to generation. They are hidden primordial images or '*archetypes*' which represents the memories of race. As they are deeply unconscious, they are expressed in mythology, dreams, motifs and hallucinations. Surprisingly, themes and symbols of the above resembles very much in each individual, thereby providing ample proof of unity of human consciousness. Most of the Religions are meant for explaining and ordering the world, the reality and has very piotal role to play in developing the moral fibre and consciousness of mankind.

If truth is the real liberation, and one find it difficult to get it in the realm of philosophy and religion, the reality should be searched somewhere else. There must be some fundamental truth about the universe. *Physics* deals with space, time, matter, energy and its domain is the entire universe from beginning to end. However nothing is fixed there also. The irony today is that physics has reached a stage where there isn't any single description of the universe. They keep reconstructing universes in order to explain the same phenomena. Once considered as the end limit, the classical physics of Newtonion Laws collapsed. Atom got Fragmented and Quantum physics, theory of relativity and complementarity replaced the earlier understanding. In Einstein's relativity theory, the conventional attributes of mass, length, energy and time lose their absolute significance, whereas, in Niels Bohr's complementarity theory the conventional attributes of waves and particles lose their absolute significance. Quantum mechanics had held the particle-wave duality whereas, de Broglie, a French Prince, demonstrated in 1924 that an electron is both a particle and a wave. A step further, Werner Heisenberg in 1927 stated with proof that no events, even the atomic events can be described with any certainty. There are aspects of reality about which nothing definite can be said.

There is no fixed, absolute truth about the physical universe, as was assumed earlier in the Newtonian Physics.

It would soon be discovered, too, that they are relative also to the observer who observed them. In 1927 John Von Neymann wrote in his book 'The Mathematical Foundations of Quantum Theory' that the most important component in an experiment is the human consciousness of the observer. A step further, In 1972 Alain Aspect performed an experiment on 'twin' atoms in which he found that two atoms separated by a large distance seem to communicate with each other. This take place in no time and without any physical means. Communication, so far being understood as property of mind only, seems to be present in physical entities too. All these led us to believe with some evidence that there is but one universal consciousness that pervades all of creations.

Philosophy, religion and science attempt to provide knowledge about universal consciousness. Knowledge is necessary but not sufficient condition for development of human consciousness. In fact knowledge at any given time manifests truth only partially and violence in the world has increased with the expansion of knowledge. What is required is right will and freedom from wrong perception of self and others. Whereas, philosophy, religion and science talks about consciousness in a theoretical way, it is the Yoga which provides the actual technology for its real development. With the aid of Yoga technology, when something of subject's immediate purpose is achieved, he is free to upgrade his purpose to the ultimate achievable–the realization of truth itself. Yoga submits that what is usually achieved by normal pace can be multiplied one hundred fold by recourse to Yoga technology for improvement of both the body and mind. Yoga believes that the problem of man is man and that everything done for him, outside of him, is mere artificial conditioning and not real. Man is the cause of his own bondage or freedom. By experience and practice, we all have realized this. Yoga is an integrated, holistic system of self culture which aims at the harmonious development and health of the body-mind complex. It have 1. Conditioned personal-social behaviour (Yama), 2. Yoga attitude (niyama), 3. Physical discipline (āsana), 4. Control over bionergy (prāṇāyāma), 5. Abstraction (pratyāhārā), 6. Concentration (dhāranā), 7. Meditation (dhyāna), and 8. Consciousness absolute (Samadhi).

At its highest culmination, the yoga technology ends with the liberation and realization of self, and helps to develop universal consciousness, there by facilitates to overcome individual and societal violence.

To conclude Advaita Vedanta emphasises that the 'consciousness is one, omnipotent and omnipresent' the truth is one and wise call it by different name.

References

1. Maslow, A.H., Toward a Psychology of being, Princeton, N.J. : Van Nostrand, 1962 (2nd ed., 1968).

The Classical Yoga of Patanjali

Ganesh Shankar

Yoga has already become very popular amongst the masses all over the world. However, for this very reason, many quacks and charlatans are exploiting masses for their selfish goals and due to them very queer notions regarding Yoga have become prevalent among people. Some consider yoga as a set of exercises for maintaining health, others consider it as some mysterious means of getting supernatural powers, whereas still others think it to be a means of getting a kick from sensory experience and entering into extra sensory perception. We can find a number of popular books on yoga in street book stalls all over the world. The titles such as "Yoga for Youth", "Yoga and sex", "Yoga for beauty etc. speak for themselves. Of course, yoga has something to do with all these things but by isolating an aspect and laying undue stress on the same, misguiding picture of yoga has been presented in such books. Moreover, these books do not represent and sound study of the ancient text on yoga.

The yoga system handed down under the name of Patanjali and presented in the slender volume of his Yoga Sutra (which, however, is practically always edited together with bulky commentaries) has gained the reputation of being the classical exposition of Yoga. It is sometimes referred to as Raja Yoga, which can be translated as the royal path. Patanjali's Yoga is the second of the systematic or integral expositions of the Yoga technique that have been preserved from ancient times. It is possible to say that upon the whole it is more elaborate and summarises the actual technique of Yoga procedures more exactly than the Buddhist exposition. This is probably due to the fact that Patanjali's Yoga Sutra are of the nature of a technical manual, whereas the Buddhist exposition is incorporated in live discourses of the Buddha with his disciple. As to the time and the personality of the author of the Yoga Sutra, full agreement has not yet been reached among scholars because of the lack of decisive evidence and the scarcity of reliable material on which to base definite views. Virtually nothing is known about Patanjali himself, and not even legendary date have been handed down. In this respect the difference between him and the creator of the first integral Yoga system, the Buddha, cannot be greater. There are other obvious differences, too. The Buddha was the founder of his system, the Buddha cannot be greater. There are other obvious differences, too. The Buddha was the founder of his system, even though, admittedly, he made use of some of the experiences he had previously gained under various yoga teachers of the time. Patanjali was neither a founder nor a leader of a new movement or community and his personality in no way emerges from his text, which is very short, condensed and impersonal. On analysis we see that he did not aim at creating anything new. The ingenuity of his achievement lies in the thoroughness and completeness with which all the important stages of yoga practice and mental experiences are included in his scheme. Patanjali was a codifier of what was best in the Yoga practice and knowledge of his time. His time cannot, however, be determined with any degree of accuracy. He was certainly post-Buddhist, although views have been expressed to the contrary and it is hardly possible to place him much before the starting-point of our era, although some place him several centuries later. From various discussions of the problem the resulting impression is that the composition of Patanjali's Yoga Sutra could have taken place any time between 300 B.C. and 300 A.D. what is beyond doubt, however, is that the material the sutras contain dates back before this period and some of it even before the time of the Buddha. There are probably also or two later interpolations in the text of the Sutras, particularly in its polemical part, which can be dated to the fourth or fifth century A.D. Some authors also have made it seem most likely that the text of the Sutras is not a unitary work, but combines into one whole two or even three originally separate texts. This again only confirms that the final redactor of the text, whoever he was, was not and did not intend to be an original author of a new teaching, but simply created a systematic presentation of the Yoga of his time.

The methodical scheme of Patanjali's Yoga has–like that of the Buddha–eight part. All of them had been known before Patanjali and their gradual emergence and even the process of ordering them into a sequence almost identical with that of the Yoga Sutra can be followed in the Yoga Upanisads. The Yoga Upanisads do not belong to the group of the oldest Brahmanical Upanisadic texts in which mythology, symbology and philosophical speculation are combined with a kind of metaphysical vision, sometimes based on meditational absorption (dhyana–Chand, Up.VII, 6, i), but their contents are based on an equally old tradition, which developed in the main outside the brahmanical circles in the communities and schools of non-orthodox ascetics. As the Brahmanical quest for the experience of the Ultimate grew important, at least in some quarters, and found acceptance among spiritually-minded Brahmans as being higher than the practice of traditional sacrifices, the independent Yoga tradition penetrated more and more into the Upanisads, the Svetasvatara and Katha being the best illustrations of this trend. There are even sections of these Upanisads already describing the Yoga path or practice, which gradually acquires a systematic form. For instance, Katha Upanisad mentions the basic requirements of Yoga practice, such as the withdrawal of the mind's attention from the senses (pratyahara) and the training in the concentration of the mind (dharana) with the subsequent unification of the mind with the ultimate reality (samadhi) Even different stages of samadhi are described. Svetasvatara Upanisad is even more explicit in its description of the Yoga path, although it is not presented systematically there. But it even mentions physical constituents of yoga practice : asana (position) and pranayama (regulation of breathing), in addition to the mental ones: pratyahara, dharna, dhyana and samadhi. Those subsequent Upanisads that specialise in yoga and are therefore known as yoga upanisads elaborate on various aspects of yoga practice and deal also with philosophical and religious elements that often accompany yoga practice, according to the school to which each particular Upanisad belongs. The yoga sutras of Patanjali appeared during a time when yoga was no longer the practice of a few but had become very popular as a result of the spread of Buddhism, Jainism, and other unorthodox religious circles who modified yoga practice and interpretation to suit their respective sectarian cults and beliefs. This led inevitably to the loosening of some strict yoga rules and principles of practice. In particular the principle of the purification of the mind as a preparation for a higher spiritual vision was too much influenced by sectarian ideas and imagery and the goal became the achievement of ecstatic union with one's chosen deity (ista devata). This in turn led in some cases to a less strict observance of the moral discipline current in ascetic and yoga schools, and in extreme cases even led to its obliteration. In this situation Patanjali's text set standards for the practice and aims of yoga which while allowing some space for different conceptions of the nature of existence, the final goal and the role, if any, of God in yoga were so impressive and found such strong consensus that they could not easily be disregarded. The yoga sutras therefore came to be viewed as a classical text of yoga and have remained so practically till the present day. They represent the strict, sober and sincere trend in Yoga as it was followed by generations of earnest truth-seekers over many centuries, a trend that had previously found expression only in the Buddha's eightfold path, from which Patanjali obviously benefited. His eightfold path can be summarised as under:

1. **Yama:** This word may be interpreted as "abstinence." It represents the conscious endeavour on the part of the Yogi to abstain from doing things that keep his mind involved in the indiscriminate struggle for survival and satisfaction within the existing scale of values in life. Although the stress seems to lie on abstaining, which is a negative concept the contents of the "abstinences" are sometimes positive. They are five in number:

(*a*) Ahimsa–means non-violence, abstaining from killing and hurting other beings.

(*b*) Satya–is truthfulness and implies abstaining from telling lies and from falseness of any kind.

(*c*) Asteya–means abstaining from stealing.

(*d*) Brahmcarya–literally "divine faring" means living in accordance with the standards of the goal of yoga, which is union with God or with the ultimate reality, or the final direct knowledge thereof (depending on interpretation). Therefore those associations that imide progress towards the goal owing to the overwhelming impact they may have on the mind and the whole personality have to renounced. Sexual union has been regarded as the most powerful fiverting influence of this kind and has therefore been avoided by serious fully committed yogis. Brahmacarya therefore become synonymous with chastity or celibacy.

(*e*) Aparigraha–may be interpreted as "abstaining from appropriating." It is an attitude of mind that does not consider anything to be one's own, even if one is using it (such as the physical body) and even if it seems to be essential for life (including "one's own" life).

2. **Niyama:** Both yama and niyama are words derived from the same root "yam" which as a verb means to control, to tame. Niyama can be interpreted as "observance" and it represents the yogi's progressive effort to observe certain principles that prepare his personality for achievements of a higher order. They are also five in number which are summarised as follows:

(*a*) Sauca–means purity and it is external as well as internal. The yogi has to strive for pure thinking, speaking and acting , to keep his body clean, see to the purity of his food, act from pure motives and cleanse his mind of sensuality and urges.

(*b*) Santosa–is contentment. It expresses the willingness of the yogi to accept and face reality as it is without being elated or depressed by it. He has to bear equally pleasure and pain, gain and loss, fame and contempt, success and failure, sympathy and hostility. He must be able, if necessary, to reduce his needs to the bare necessities of life.

(c) Tapas–means traditionally "austerity" and introduces into the practices of yoga forbearance, fasts and other ascetic practices that help to reduce the yogi's dependence on things that cannot be altogether avoided, but should not become desirable for their own sake. In this way he increases his self control.

(d) Svadhyaya–is self development of self education and points to the necessity of continuous study, constant learning and development of one's intelligence and higher mental faculties.

(e) Isvarapranidhana–may be interpreted as "constant thought of divine" (a more literal rendering is "surrender to the Lord"). It is an admonition to constantly aware that there is the transcendent, which the yogi may not yet have experienced, but which is his goal and which should therefore be constantly in his mind, accompanying all his thoughts and actions.

3. **Asana:** Asana means "position", "posture." For efficient yoga practice it is essential to be able to assume a stable and agreeable position when training the mind so that the mind is free from bodily interference, which normally compels one to move or change position. In India since time immemorial it has been a cross-legged position. It has several varieties of which the lotus posture (Padmasana) is the most impressive one.

4. **Pranayama:** Pranayama is the control of the process of breathing. It is usually done in the position chosen for yoga practice. It regulates breathing and its rhythm, especially by showing down and also by introducing longer breaks between the phases of breathing. Since there is a close connection between the flow of respiration and the dynamics of the mind, the help which can thereby be obtained in

establishing some balance of mind, enhancing its clarity and capacity for observation, is considerable.

5. **Pratyahara**: It means "withdrawal." It is the first purely mental step in this system of yoga, aiming as it does not at preparing the mind for spiritual vision, which can come from within only when the mind becomes receptive in that direction rather than expecting everything to enter if from outside in a similar way to all the information about the external world. A mind made clear and calm by pranayama is now further purified by withdrawing its attention from the activity of the senses, which normally constantly fill it with images derived from external objects. The withdrawal of attention from the senses cuts off the flow of perceptions created by external objects and the mind can then be trained in the succeeding steps of the path, which involve the technique of opening it to inner vision.

6. **Dharana:** It means concentration and its aim is to bring about "one-pointedness" (ekagrata) of the mind, which can they stay focused on one particular object of its (internal) experience in a way unknown to the mind when it operates on the level of sense data. This concentration also results in a degree of understanding and comprehension of the chosen object that eventually penetrates into its very essence or nature.

7 **Dhyana:** It may be translated as contemplation or absorption. It is reached when concentration becomes spontaneous. It is then a natural process for the mind of the yogi, just as thinking is natural for everybody else, so that no special effort needed to embark on it. At this stage the penetration of the essence of the object of contemplation becomes complete. This technique then enables the mind to approach reality as such "from inside" which is the suprasensory and supra intellectual direct way of cognition. This leads to the final achievement.

8. **Samadhi**: It is translated as unification. Samadhi is the crown of yoga endeavours in Patanjali's system. It is the fully conscious and "factual" unification of the Yogi's vision or cognitive capacity or mind itself with the heart of reality

in its wholeness which sets him free. He reaches final liberation from the bondage to limited forms of existence that can exist only through ignorance or lack of total vision. But samadhi is not a simple experience. It is realised in stages. The sequence and relationship of these stages is not entirely clear from Patanjali's text. It is also quite possible that in practice the stages cannot be fully distinguished from one another and that they are simply a broad guide for the yogi to measure his progress approximately before he reaches the final goal. However, some tentative picture of the stages of progress through samadhi has to be given.

References

1. Bhushan, L.I. (1997), "Yoga psychology–A re-emerging field", Yoga–Sivananda Math 8:4:13-26.
2. Jacobi, C.P., "On the original system of Yoga, Eng. translation by Prof. R.D. Vedekar, YM Vol. XV.
3. Kenghe, C.T. (1975), "Yoga As Depth-Psychology & Para-Psychology," Bharat Manisha, Varanasi, Vol. I.
4. Karambelkar, P.V. (1987), "Patanjali Yoga Sutra" Kaivalyadhama, Lonavla.

   Saraswati, Swami Niranjanananda (1993), "Yoga Darshan", Sri Panchdarshanam, Paramhansa Alakh Bara, Rikhia, Deoghar Bihar.
5. Saraswati, Swami Satyananda (1980), "Yoga from shore to shore (3rd edition) Bihar School of Yoga, Munger (Bihar).

महर्षि पतंजलि और आचार्य बुद्धघोष की योग साधनाऐं

पिंकी भनोट एवं सुरेन्द्र सिंह नेगी

योग दर्शन साधना का दर्शन है। अत: वह एक मार्ग है और इस अर्थ में वह बुद्ध के मार्ग से एक बड़ी समानता रखता है, किन्तु फिर भी उसकी तात्विक परिस्थिति बौद्ध दर्शन के समान न होकर सांख्य दर्शन की ही है। विभिन्न तात्विक परिस्थितियों के होते हुये भी दो दर्शन अपने साधना मार्ग में कितने समान हो सकते हैं इसका अनुत्तर उदाहरण हमें बौद्ध दर्शन और योग दर्शन में मिलता है।

जिस प्रकार समग्र बुद्ध शासन चार आर्य सत्यों पर प्रतिष्ठित है[1] उसी प्रकार योग मार्ग भी दुख, समुदाय, निरोध मार्ग इस चतुर्विध समस्या के विभाजन को लेकर ही प्रवृत्त होता है। उसका मन्तव्य है कि यह संसार दुख, बहुल है अत: हेय है फिर वह कहता है कि प्रधान पुरुष का संयोग ही हेय का हेतु है अत: उस संयोग की आत्यन्तिक निवृत्ति ही हान है और साम्यदर्शन ही हानोपाय है[2]। सांख्यकार का विचार है कि उपर्युक्त प्रकार से दुख की निवृत्ति ''दृष्ट'' पदार्थों के द्वारा संभव नहीं है[3]। इनसे तो दुखों का तांता लगा ही रहेगा। यदि एक बार इनसे दुख हठ भी जायेंगे तो फिर उनकी अनुवृत्ति होना आवश्यक है[4]। दुख का सम्यक् निरोध तो तभी हो सकता है जब अविद्या के बीज दग्ध कर दिये जायें जिससे कि उनमें से दुख के कुलहे फिर उपज ही न सकें। सांख्याचार्यो का एक उद्‌घोष यह भी है कि ''दृष्ट'' से तो दुख की आत्यान्तिक निवृत्ति हो ही नहीं सकती, वह ''आनुश्राविक'' से भी होना असंभव है[5]। वैदिक कर्मकाण्ड हमें बचा नहीं सकता। वह तो स्वयं ''अविशुद्धि'' ''क्षय'' और ''अतिशय'' ये युक्त है[6]। उस वैदिक कर्मकाण्ड का विपरीत मार्ग ही श्रेयान है। कौन सा विपरीत मार्ग? वही जो ''व्यक्त'' (महाभूत) ''अव्यक्त'' (प्रधान) प्रकृति और

पुरूष के ज्ञान से निष्पन्न होता है। वैदिक कर्मकाण्ड का यह निश्चय ही अत्यन्त तीव्र प्रतिवाद है[7]। इतनी दूर तो संभवत: बुद्ध भी नहीं गये। ''श्रेयान'' शब्द को लेकर मक्समूलर ने यह दिखलाने का प्रयत्न किया है कि वहां वैदिक कर्मकाण्ड की अपेक्षा में ही प्रकृति पुरूष विषयक विज्ञान की श्रेष्ठता दिखाई गई है अत: तद्विपरीत: श्रेयान''। कहने का तात्पर्य यह है कि उसके विपरीत जो है वह अधिक अच्छा है और वैसे वैदिक कर्मकाण्ड भी अच्छा है[8]। यदि सांख्याचार्य को इतना समन्वय ही अपेक्षित होता तो वे वैदिक कर्मकाण्ड को ''अविशुद्धि'' ''क्षय'' और अतिशय से युक्त कभी नहीं बतलाते फिर भी सांख्य दर्शन की सत्य के ज्ञापक के रूप में वेद में श्रद्धा है।

बौद्ध दर्शन सृष्टि की उत्पत्ति के विषय को लेकर अधिकांश में प्रवृत्त नहीं होता फिर भी बौद्ध दर्शन की दृष्टि को निरूपित करना आवश्यक है। सबसे पहले सृष्टि के विकास की श्रेणी में हम देखते हैं कि ''प्रधान'' रूप ''मूल प्रवृत्ति'' है जिसका फिर और कोई मूल नहीं है। इस दृष्टिकोण से देखने पर निश्चय ही यह प्रलोभन हो सकता है कि यह ''मूल प्रकृति'' कहीं उस बौद्ध ''अविद्या'' से तो संबंध या समानता नहीं रखती जो ''प्रतीत्य समुत्पाद'' के सबसे पहले प्रत्यय के रूप में स्मरण की जाती है और जिसके आगे प्राणियों के पूर्व कोटि का पता नहीं चलता। ''प्रतीत्य समुत्पाद'' का उपदेश कारणवाद की समस्या को हल करने के लिए नहीं दिया गया[9]। अत: उस रूप में उसकी समानता भी किसी अन्य सिद्धान्त से नहीं की जा सकती। बौद्ध अविद्या को हमें सांख्य के प्रधान से कभी मिलाने के विभ्रम में नहीं पड़ना चाहिये इसके लिए हमें आचार्य बुद्धघोष ने बहुत पहले ही आगाह कर दिया है। अपने ''विशुद्धिमग्ग'' ग्रन्थ में इन ''अट्ठकथाचरिय'' ने सांख्य योग के प्रकृति और पुरूष के द्वैतवाद का प्रत्यायान किया है और प्रकृतिवासियों की ''मूल प्रकृति'' से ''अविज्जा'' की समानता दिखाने का बड़ा विरोध किया है[10]। घरिणामिनिस्यत्व'' का भाव सांख्य विकास वाद में निहित है वही नित्य समुत्पन्न और नित्य निरूद्ध होने वाले बौद्ध धर्म में भी है और जैसा कि यह देखा गया है कि दोनों में ही उनके प्रति ''आनात्भाव'' करने में ही कल्याण का मार्ग माना गया है, बौद्ध दर्शन में तो प्रतीत्य समुत्पन्न पंच स्कन्धों में और सांख्य दर्शन में ''परिणामानिनित्य'' प्रकृति के विचारों में। कतं ने जो बौद्ध ''अविद्या'' की समता सांख्य ''प्रधान से, संस्कारों की समता बुद्धि से, विज्ञान की समता अहंकार से, नामरूप की समता तन्मात्राओं से, षड़ायन इन्द्रियों से और समग्र ''प्रतीत्य समुत्पाद'' की समता सांख्योक्त ''प्रत्ययसंघ से दिखाने का प्रस्ताव किया है उसे ठीक नहीं समझना चाहिए जब तक कि यह न देख लिया जाये कि सांख्य दर्शन में ''बुद्धि-अहंकार, तन्मात्राऐं

और इन्द्रियां किन अर्थों में प्रयुक्त की गई हैं, तब तक हम यह नहीं कह सकते कि क्रमश: बौद्ध दर्शन में निरूपित ''संस्कार विज्ञान'' ''नामरूप'' और षडायतनों से उनका क्या संबंध है[11]। भारतीय दर्शन में मनोविज्ञान की दृष्टि से दो ही दर्शन सबसे अधिक महत्वपूर्ण हैं, बौद्धदर्शन और सांख्य योग दर्शन जिन्होंने प्राय: औपनिषद मनोविज्ञान को ही एक व्यवस्थित व्यरूप प्रदान किया है जिसे अन्य-आस्तिक'' दर्शनों ने भी बिना किसी विवाद के अपने प्रयोजनों के लिये प्रयुक्त किया है। सबसे पहले चक्षुरादि इन्द्रियां स्थूल कारण या साधन है। ये इन्द्रिय संस्कारों को केन्द्र की ओर ले जाने के लिये इन्द्रियों को प्रदान करती हैं तब मन, इन्द्रियों तथा बाह्य साधनों अर्थात् भौतिक नेत्र, श्रोत आदि से संयुक्त होता है। मन उन संस्कारों की ओर आगे बढ़ाता है एवं उन्हें बुद्धि के सामने उपस्थित करता है। बुद्धि उन पर विचार करती है उनका अवगाहन करती है इसके पश्चात् यह सब क्रिया-प्रतिक्रिया पुरूष के सम्मुख उपस्थित होती है जो ज्ञान का वास्तविक अधिष्ठान है। बुद्धि जब ठीक निर्णय कर लेती है तो उसे कार्यान्वित करने के लिये मन को दे देती है[12]। मन पाँच कर्मेन्द्रियों के द्वारा बुद्धि के निश्चयों का पालन करता है यही संक्षेपत: योग-मनोविज्ञान है इस विषय में सबसे महत्वपूर्ण बात जो बौद्धदर्शन के साथ तुलनात्मक अध्ययन करते समय हमें याद रखनी चाहिये, वह यह है कि प्रकृति और पुरूष के द्रष्टा और दृश्य के जड़ और चैतन्य के संबंध को भली-भांति से समझने के लिए ही सांख्य ने अपने मनोविज्ञान का विधान किया है ताकि प्रकृति और उसके विकारों की प्रतिच्छाया से पुरूष उसमें ''अहं'' की भावना न करने लगे, ताकि प्रकृति के ही संसरण बंधन और मोक्ष में वह अपना संसरण, बन्धन और मोक्ष न मानने लगे इसलिये परमर्षि ने यह सब ''पुरूषार्थ हेतुक'' ''निमित्त नैमित्तक'' प्रसंग कहा है और इसलिये इन सभी मनोवैज्ञानिक क्रिया प्रतिक्रियाओं के मूल में होकर उन्हें कहना पड़ा है: ''पुरूषार्थ एक हेतुर्न केनचित् कार्यते करणम्''[13]। हम बुद्ध के द्वारा निरूपित समग्र विज्ञान में ''चित्त चैतसिक'' और ''रूप'' के रूप में अथवा ''कुशल'' ''अकुशल'' और अव्याकृत के भागों में तो बंटा देखते हैं और नदी के स्रोत की तरह उनका बहना भी देखते हैं जिनमें ''अहं'' बुद्धि कभी न करने का भगवान बुद्ध ने उपदेश दिया किन्तु पुरूषार्थ एवं हेतु. जैसी कोई आवाज हम वहां कदाचित नहीं सुनते। वहां तो ''एवं पन्चस्कन्ध-युकिं लब्धं किं हसं खेत'' ऐसी ही साधना की ध्वनि की प्रधानता है। सांख्य योग का दृष्टिकोण अधिक संग्रहात्मक है किन्तु उसमें व्यावहारिकता कम है और बौद्ध दुष्टिकोण जब कि नैतिक अभिव्याप्ति से अपने मनोविज्ञान को ओत-प्रोत कर देता है न तो चित्त चैतसिकों के प्रतीत्य समुत्पन्न भाव को ही वह सत्य का अंतिम स्वरूप मानने की ओर प्रस्ताव सा करता जान पड़ता है, जैसा कि संभवत: नहीं है।

सांख्य-योग मतानुसार सर्गक्रम का विशद विवेचन करने के बाद ही सांख्यकारिका में यह महत्वपूर्ण कारिका आती है। ''इत्येव प्रकृति मध्दाभि विशेषभूत पर्यन्तः। प्रतिपुरूष विमोक्षार्थ स्वार्थ इव परार्थ आरंभ''[14]। यहां हमें केवल इत्येष प्रकृतिकृतों इतने से ही तात्पर्य है। जब एक बार सर्गक्रम निरूपण में सांख्याचार्य प्रवृत्त हुये तो निश्चय ही उन्हें इसका तो उत्तर देना ही था कि आखिर यह सब किया किसने है। बुद्ध तो सर्ग आदि के प्रश्नों में ही नहीं पड़े बल्कि उस विषयक जिज्ञासा को ही उन्होंने असंगत जिज्ञासा कहा और केवल दुख की आत्यान्तिक निवृत्ति के मार्ग का ही आचरण करने को कहा किन्तु सांख्याचार्य जिन्होंनें दुख की निवृत्ति के लिए व्यक्ताव्यक्तज्ञ विज्ञान को ही परम श्रेयान मार्ग माना है तो फिर वे उसके उत्तर देने में तथागत की तरह उदासीनता कैसे धारण कर सकते थे। तथागत के लिए तो चाहे यह ''प्रकृति कृत'' हो तब भी और चट्टान हो तब भी, चाहे ईश्वर कृत हो या न हो तब भी, चाहे ब्रह्मकृत हो या न हो, तब भी परम आश्वासन है। पतंजलि के योग सूत्र में ईश्वर प्रणिधान का वैकल्पिक महत्व बताया गया है[15]। ईश्वर प्रणिधान को भगवान पतंजलि ने समाधि की प्राप्ति में सहायक माना है और उसको ''पुरूष विशेष'' कह कर परिभाषित किया है, उसमें निकतिशय सर्वज्ञ बीज का होना बताया है, पूर्वजों का भी उसे गुरू बताया है और उसके वाचक प्रणव के जप और उसके अर्थ भावना से दिखाई प्रत्येक चेतना के अधिगम एवं योग के मार्ग में सभी अन्तरायों के अभाव में संभावना। अतः उनके क्रियायोग में तपस और स्वाध्याय के साथ ईश्वर-प्रणिधान ने भी एक आवश्यक स्थान पाया है[16]। बुद्ध ने इसके बिना ही अपना काम चला लिया है।

संदर्भ सूची

(1) बौद्ध तथा अन्य भारतीय दर्शन-प्रथम भाग, प्रकरण-4 पृष्ठ-195।

(2) व्यास भाष्य-2/15।

(3) सा० का०-1/1।

(4) सा० का०-1/2।

(5) सा० का०-2।

(6) सा० ह्यक्शिुद्धिमग्यातिशयमुक्तः।

(7) सा० प्रवचन सूत्र-3/84।

(8) सोवनी. ए क्रिटीकल स्टडी आफ दि सांख्य सिरहम, पृ०-15।

(9) भरत सिंह उपाध्याय, ''बौद्ध तथा अन्य भारतीय दर्शन'' चतुर्थ प्रकरण पृ०-373।

(10) भरत सिंह उपाध्याय "बौद्ध तथा अन्य भारतीय दर्शन" चतुर्थ प्रकरण पृ० - 405।

(11) मेनअल आफ इण्डियन बुद्धिज्म पृ० - 47 ददरकतं, 691।

(12) सा० का० - 35 - 37।

(13) सा० का० - 31।

(14) सा० का० - 56।

(15) यो० सू० - 1/23।

(16) यो० सू० - 2/1।

चित्त प्रसादन के उपाय

ईश्वर भारद्वाज एवं रीता भल्ला

महर्षि पतन्जलि ने योगसूत्र में योग की परिभाषा करते हुए कहा है–"योगश्चित्तवृत्तिनिरोधः"[1] अर्थात् चित्त की वृत्तियों का निरोध करना योग है। उन्होंने चित्तवृत्ति निरोध के विभिन्न उपायों की भी चर्चा की है जैसे–अभ्यास-वैराग्य[2], अष्टांग योग[3], क्रियायोग[4] आदि। ये उपाय योगाभ्यास में जिन साधकों की गति है, उनके लिए सहज हो सकते हैं। नए साधक को अथवा सामान्य लोगों के लिए ये साधन सहजग्राह्य नहीं हैं। चित्त (मन) कितना बलवान है? यह तो स्वयं भगवान कृष्ण ने गीता में स्पष्ट कर दिया है कि मन निश्चय ही चंचल और कठिनाई से वश में आने वाला है किन्तु इसे अभ्यास और वैराग्य द्वारा वश में किया जा सकता है[5]। अभ्यास वैराग्य श्रेष्ठ साधकों के लिए है। साधारण व्यक्ति अथवा नवीन साधक को बिना मन को वश में किए योग मार्ग में बढ़ना अत्यन्त कठिन कार्य है। यह तो मन को वश में करने वाले साधक को ही प्राप्त हो सकता है[6]। इसलिए सर्वप्रथम साधक को चाहिए कि चित्त को निर्मल करें। चित्त को निर्मल करने के लिए शोधन क्रियाओं[7] का अभ्यास करें। इसके साथ ही निम्नलिखित उपायों का आश्रय लेकर चित्त को प्रसन्न रखें, तभी वह योग की स्थिति के लिए उपयुक्त होगा। चित्त प्रसादन हेतु किया गया प्रयास भी योग मार्ग के लिए साधन ही है।

1. ईश्वर प्रणिधान

ईश्वर-प्रणिधान ईश्वर के प्रति पूर्ण समर्पण का भाव है। शरीर, इन्द्रिय, मन, प्राण, समस्त कर्म, वासनाएँ, कर्मफल भावनाएँ आदि सभी को ईश्वर के प्रति समर्पित कर देना ही ईश्वर प्रणिधान है। यह समझना कि जो कुछ भी शुभाशुभ कर्म फलेच्छा या निष्काम भाव से मैं करता हूँ, वह सभी आपको (परमेश्वर को) अर्पित करता हूँ[8]। स्वयं भगवान कृष्ण ने कार्म-भोजन, यज्ञ, दानादि अपने को अर्पित करने का आदेश दिया है[9]। इस प्रकार ब्रह्म को अर्पित किए गए कर्म का फल कर्ता को नहीं मिलता और वह जल में कमल के पत्ते की तरह उससे अलग

ही रहता है[10]। सामान्य स्थिति में भी देखा जाए तो सब कुछ शुभाशुभ परमात्मा को अर्पित करने के बाद व्यक्ति निश्चिंत हो जाता है। ऐसा साधक योग मार्ग पर चलने के उपयुक्त हो जाता है तथा प्रसन्न रहता है।

2. प्रणव – जाप

परमेश्वर को सर्वोत्तम नाम ''प्रणव'' या ''ओम्'' कहा गया है[11]। ओम् को ''ब्रह्म'' और ''सब कुछ'' कहा गया है[12]। उस ओंकार रूपी धनुष पर आत्मा रूपी वाण को चढ़ाकर ब्रह्म रूपी लक्ष्य को प्राप्त करना चाहिए[13]। प्रणव – जाप करके भी चित्त में प्रसन्नता आती है। जाप करते समय उसके अर्थ का चिन्तन भी करना चाहिए[14]। चित्त तभी स्थिर होता है। क्लेश, कर्म, संस्कार, भावना, वासना सभी धुल जाते हैं तथा चित्त निर्मल हो जाता है। जिससे प्रसन्नता बनी रहती है। निज स्वरूप के साक्षात्कार के साथ – साथ सम्पूर्ण विघ्नों का नाश भी हो जाता है[15]।

3. एकतत्वाभ्यास

व्याधि आदि नौ विघ्नों (अन्तरायों) तथा दुःखादि विक्षेपों को दूर करने के लिए एकतत्वाभ्यास का विधान किया गया है[16]। एकतत्व के अभ्यास से तात्पर्य है–इष्ट का बार – बार ध्यान करने का प्रयास। इसके लिए जिस वस्तु, पदार्थ, व्यक्ति, देव प्रतिमा आदि से साधक सर्वाधिक श्रद्धा व प्रेम भाव रखता है, वही उसका अभिमत (इष्ट) होना चाहिए। ऐसा करने से एकाग्रता बढ़ेगी और विक्षेपों का नाश हो जाएगा। इस प्रकार चित्त में प्रसन्नता का संचरण होगा।

4. भावना

राग, ईर्ष्या, परोपकार – चिकीर्षा, असूया, द्वेष व अमर्ष–ये छह कालुष्य चित्त को मलिन तथा दुःखी करते हैं। इनके कारण साधना में अग्रसर होना असंभव है। इन कालुष्यों को दूर करने के लिए मैत्री, करूणा, मुदिता और उपेक्षा की भावना का आश्रय लेना चाहिए। सुखी, दुःखी, पुण्यात्मा और पापियों के लिए क्रमशः मैत्री, करूणा, मुदिता और उपेक्षा की भावना रखने से चित्त प्रसन्न रहता है[17]।

सुखी व्यक्ति को देखकर मनुष्य अपने ईर्ष्या – कालुष्य के कारण दुःखी रहता है। ऐसा सुख मुझे क्यों नहीं प्राप्त है? उस सुख को प्राप्त करने की इच्छा उसे कष्ट देती है। यदि व्यक्ति उस सुखी व्यक्ति से मित्रता कर ले तो वह राग तथा ईर्ष्या – कालुष्य से बच सकता है। मित्र के सुख में अपना सुख समझकर राग से तथा मित्र के लाभ में अपना लाभ समझकर ईर्ष्या से बच सकता है। इसी

प्रकार दु:खी व्यक्ति को देखकर यदि उसके प्रति करूणा का भाव हृदय में उत्पन्न हो जाए तो व्यक्ति परोपकार-चिकीर्षा (दूसरे का बुरा करने की इच्छा) से बच सकता है। उस दु:खी व्यक्ति के स्थान पर स्वयं को समझकर उसके कष्ट का अनुभव करना चाहिए।

पुण्यात्मा को देखकर हम उसमें दोष देखते हैं कि इस व्यक्ति ने दानादि धार्मिक कृत्य अपने नाम के लिए किए हैं अथवा इसने गलत रीति से धनार्जन करके यह कार्य किया है। यदि उसको देखकर हम प्रसन्नता से यह कहें कि बहुत अच्छा कार्य किया है, परमात्मा इसकी और उन्नति करे, इसका कल्याण करे तो इससे असूया-कालुष्य की निवृत्ति होती है।

पापाचारी व्यक्ति को देखकर सभी द्वेष तथा अमर्ष से भर जाते हैं। उसको सबक सिखाने के लिए तत्पर हो उठते हैं। यदि पानी को देखकर यह सोचें कि वह स्वयं अपने लिए बुरा कर रहा है, मैं क्यों स्वयं को दूषित करूँ? शासन स्वयं व्यवस्था हेतु इसका उपाय करेगा, आदि। इस भावना से चित्त में विक्षोम नहीं होगा तथा द्वेष व अमर्ष कालुष्य दूर हो जाएंगे।

उपर्युक्त भावनाओं से चित्त में प्रसन्नता आएगी तथा चित्त एकाग्रता की स्थिति को प्राप्त कर लेगा।

5. प्रच्छर्दन व विधारण

प्राणवायु को दोनों नासापुटों से बाहर निकालकर बाह्य कुंभक करना भी चित्त को स्थिरता की स्थिति देता है[18]। श्वास को रोकने पर चित्तकी चंचलता भी समाप्त हो जाती है[19]। चित्त मलों का प्राणायाम के अभ्यास द्वारा शीघ्र ही नाश हो जाता है जैसे अग्नि से धातुओं के मल नष्ट हो जाते हैं[20]। ऐसा स्वच्छ चित्त प्रसन्न रहता है तथा एकाग्रता की स्थिति प्राप्त कर लेता है।

6. विषयवती प्रवृत्ति होना

शब्द, स्पर्श, रूप, रस व गन्ध में प्रवृत्ति होने से भी चित्त की स्थिति दृढ़ होती है[21]। नासिकाग्र में संयम से गन्ध, जिह्वाग्र में संयम से रस, तालु में संयम से रूप, जिह्वा मध्य में संयम से स्पर्श, जिह्वामूल में संयम से शब्द का साक्षात्कार होता है। इनमें चित्त को लगाने से (संयम से) संशय का नाश होता है तथा चित्त में प्रसन्नता आती है जिससे एकाग्रता बनती है।

7. सत्वप्रधान प्रकाशवती प्रवृत्ति

रजोगुण व तमोगुण से रहित सत्वप्रधान ज्योतिषमती प्रवृत्ति भी चित्त को स्थिर

करती है[22]। सुषुम्ना नाड़ी में स्थित चक्रों पर चित्त को स्थिर करने से भी चित्त प्रसन्न होता है और एकाग्रता आती है।

8. योगियों के चित्त का ध्यान

राग से रहित, आसक्तिरहित, चित्त वाले श्रेष्ठ योगीजनों के चित्त का ध्यान करने से भी चित्त में स्थिरता आती है[33]। क्योंकि योगियों के चित्त से सभी क्लेश, संस्कार आदि नष्ट होकर सत्व का उद्रेक रहता है। साधक उनके चित्त में संयन करता है तो वैसे ही सत्व का उद्रेक साधक के चित्त में भी हो जाता है जिससे चित्त में एकाग्रता की स्थिति आ जाती है।

9. निद्रावृत्ति का आश्रय

जाग्रतावस्था में चित रजोगुण प्रधान होने के कारण बर्हिमुख हो जाता है। निद्रा व स्वप्न की स्थिति में तमोगुण से आच्छादित होकर चित्त की वृत्तियाँ अन्तर्मुखी हो जाती हैं तथा अभाव की प्रतीति कराती हैं। यदि साधक निद्रा व स्वप्न ज्ञान का आश्रय लेकर वैसी ही अन्तर्मुखी प्रवृत्ति बनाए रखे तो चित्त स्थिर होने लगता है[24]। जैसे स्वप्न में सुन्दर, मनोहर दृश्य देखने के बाद जागने पर भी कुछ देर वैसी ही स्थिति बनी रहती है, उसी प्रकार जाग्रत होने पर भी वृत्तियों का अन्तर्मुख करने का प्रयास करना चाहिए। इससे एकाग्रता बनती है तथा चित्त प्रसन्न रहता है।

10. ध्यान

जिस व्यक्ति में अथवा वस्तु में सर्वाधिक प्रेम, श्रद्धा एवं विश्वास होता है, वही साधक के समक्ष हर समय रहती है। उसी में ध्यान लगाना सर्व सुलभ है। साधक को चाहिए कि उस प्रिय वस्तु अथवा इष्ट में ध्यान लगाने का प्रयास करे[25]। इससे चित्त में एकाग्रता आती है तथा चित्त प्रसन्न रहता है। एकाग्र हुआ चित्त किसी भी स्थल पर लगाया जा सकता है।

इन उपायों को अपनाकर चित्त को नियन्त्रित किया जा सकता है। नियन्त्रित चित्त की गति परमाणु से आकाश पर्यन्त हो जाती है[26]। इसी को चित्त की परमावश्यता कहा गया है। साधक चित्त को अपने अनुकूल चलाने में समर्थ हो जाता है। यही चित्त के प्रसादन की अवस्था है।

संदर्भ

1. योगसूत्र–1/2।
2. अभ्यास वैराग्याभ्यां तन्निरोधः/योगसूत्र–1/12।

3. यमनियमासनप्राणायामप्रत्याहारधारणाध्यानसमाधयोऽष्टावंगनि।
4. तपः स्वाध्यायेश्वरप्रणिधानानि क्रियायोगः/योगसूत्र–5/1
5. असंशयं महाबाहो मनो दुर्निग्रहं चलम्।
अभ्यासेन तु कौन्तेय वैराग्येण च गृह्यते।। गीता–6/35
6. असंयतात्मना योगो दुष्प्राप इति मे मतिः।
वश्यात्मना तुयतता शक्योअलाप्तुमुपायतः।। गीता–6/36
7. धौतिर्वस्तिस्तथानेति नौलिकी त्राटकं तथा।
कपालभातिश्चैतानि षट्कर्माणि समाचरेत्।। हठ० प्र
8. कामतोऽकामतो वापि यत् करोमि शुभाशुभम्।
तत्सर्व त्वयि संन्यस्तं त्वत्प्रयुक्तः करोम्यहम्।। गीता
9. यत्करोषि यदश्नासि यज्जुहोषि ददासि यत्।
यत्तपस्यसि कौन्तेय तत्कुरूष्व मदर्पणम्।। गीता–9/27
10. ब्रहण्याधाय कर्माणि संगं त्यक्त्वा करोति यः।
लिप्यते न स पापेन पद्मपत्रमिवाम्भसा।। गीता–5/10
11. तस्य वाचकः प्रणवः। योगसूत्र–1/27
12. ओमिति ब्रह्म। ओमितीदं सर्वम्। तैत्ति० शिक्षा०–8
13. प्रणवो धनुः रारो ह्यात्मा ब्रह्मल्लक्ष्यमुच्यते।
अप्रत्तेन वैद्धव्यं शरवत्तन्मयो भवेत्।। मुण्डको०–2/4
14. तज्जपस्तदर्धभावनम्। यो० सू०–1/28
15. ततः प्रत्यक्चेतनाधिगमोअप्यन्तरायागावश्च। यो० सू०–1/29
16. तत् प्रतिषेधार्थमेकतत्वाभ्यासः। यो० सू०–1/32
17. मैत्री करूणामुदितोपेक्षाणां सुखदुःखपुण्यापुण्यविषयाणां भावनातश्चित्तप्रसादनम्। यो० सू०–1/33
18. प्रच्छर्दनविधारणाभ्यां वा प्राणस्य/यो० सू०–1/34
19. चले वाते चलं चित्तं निश्चले निश्चलं भवेत्।
योगी स्थागुत्वमाप्नेति ततो वायुं निरोधयेत्।। ह० प्र०
20. दह्यन्ते ध्यायमानानां धातूनां हि यथा मलाः।
तथेन्द्रियाणा दह्यन्ते दोषाः प्राणस्य निग्रहात्।। मनुस्मृति
21. विषयवती वा प्रवृत्तिरूप्पन्ना मनसः स्थिति निबन्धनी। यो० सू०–1/35
22. विशोका वा ज्योतिष्मती/यो० सू०–1/36
23. वीतराग विषयं वा चित्तम्। यो० सू०–1/37
24. स्वप्ननिद्रा ज्ञानालम्बनं वा/यो० सू०–1/38
25. यथाभिमत ध्यानाद्वा/यो० सू०–1/39
26. परमाणुपरममहत्वान्तोऽस्य वशीकारः/यो० सू०–1/40

List of Contributers

Andhra Pradesh

1. Prof. P.V. Krishna Rao
   Institute for Yoga
   Andhra University
   Visakhapatnam–530 017
2. Dr. Balaiah Kovuru
   11-3-362/10/1
   Srinivasnagar
   Secunderabad–500 061

Bihar

3. Swami Niranjanananda Saraswati
   Bihar School of Yoga
   Munger–811 201

Chandigarh

4. Dr. Rakesh Kumar
   Govt. Yoga Institute
   1061/41-B
   Chandigarh–160 041

Delhi

5. Dr. S.C. Jain
   C-4/F-2, Dilshad Garden
   Delhi–110 095
6. Dr. B. Talukdar
   Deptt. of Biochemistry
   Maulana Azad Medical College
   New Delhi
7. Dr. Alka Uppal
   School of Nursing

Safdarganj Hospital
New Delhi

8. Shri Girish Jha
R-86/1, Model Town-III
First floor
Delhi–110 009

9. Shri Rameshwar Das Gupta
D-35, South Extension
Part I, *New Delhi*–110 095

10. Prof. Chandra Bhushan
Deptt. of Yoga
Gandhi Bhawan
Delhi University
Delhi

11. Vanmala Vachani
CRIY, 68, Ashoka Road
New Delhi

12. Sudha Sahni
68, CRIY, Ashoka Road
New Delhi

Haryana

13. Prof. S.P. Duggal
529/16
Panchkula–134 129

14. Dr. Narain Prakash
College of Sports
H.A.U. *Hisar*

Himachal Pradesh

15. Dr. Miss. Rita Bhalla
Deptt. of Yogic Studies
H.P. University
Shimla

Karnataka

16. Prof. B.L. Meti
Dept. of Neurophysiology
NIMHANS, *Bangalore*–560 029

Madhya Pradesh

17. Prof. R.V. Tripathi
Dept. of Sanskrit

Dr. H.S. Gour University
Sagar–470003

18. Dr. Y.S. Vagrecha
Dept. of Psychology
Dr. H.S. Gour University
Sagar–470003

19. Prof. B.K. Bandre
DirectortYoga Institute
76, Dhar Kothi, Near Robert
Nursing Home, *Indore*

20. Dr. Rajesh Shukla
5, Civil Lines
Sagar–160002

21. Dr. Mrs. Pinki Bhanot
B.D.S-1, Gour Nagar
Sagar–470003

22. Dr. S.S. Negi
Dept. of Philosophy
Dr. H.S. Gour University
Sagar–470001

23. Dr. Santosh Shukla
5, Civil Lines
Sagar

24. Dr. Ganesh Shankar
Dept. of Yogic Studies
Dr. H.S. Gour University
Sagar–470003

25. Dr. Vimla Vagrecha
University College of Education
Sagar (M.P.) 470003

Maharastra

26. Prof. M.L. Gharote (Rtd.)
A-7, Gulmohar Apartments
Bhaganwadi
Lonavla–410 402

27. Smt. Hansa Jaydeva Yogendra
The Yoga Institute
Sri Yogendra Marg, Santacruz (East)
Mumbai–400 055

28. Mr. S.V. Vyavahare
    Ghantali Mitra Mandal
    Thane–400602
29. Prof. A.N. Khodaskar, Head
    Deptt. of Yoga
    H.V.P. Mandal
    AMARAUATI (M.S.)

Meghalaya

30. Prof. K.K. Sharma
    Dept. of Education
    North Eastern Hill University
    Nehu Campus, *Shillong*–793022

Mizoram

31. Prof. K.P. Nath
    Dept. of Education
    North Eastern Hill University
    Mizoram Campus, *Aizawl*

Pondicherri

32. Yogacharini Meenakshi Devi Bhavanani
    ICYER, *Kottakuppam*–605104

Uttar Pradesh

33. Dr. Ishwar Bhardwaj
    Deptt. of Yoga
    Gurukul Kangri University
    Haridwar–249 404
34. Prof. D.N. Rai, Director
    Kundalini Yoga Institute
    Lajpat Nagar, Chowk
    Lucknow
35. Dr. Shashi Bhushan Mishra
    International Yoga Society
    Lalbag, Loni
    Ghaziabad–201102
36. Shri Harsh Vardhan Goswami
    M.M.H.P.G. College
    Ghaziabad
37. Dr. Surender Singh
    Dept. of Social Work

Lucknow University
Lucknow

38. Dr. P.D. Mishra
Dept. of Social Work
Lucknow University
Lucknow

39. Dr. Ramavtar Sharma
Rama Krishna Vivekananda Yogashrama
Aligarh

40. Dr. M. Shukla
Institute of Ophthalmology
J.N. Medical College
Aligarh Muslim University
Aligarh